Karthikeyan's

Chest X-ray Made Easy®

Karthikeyan's

Chest X-ray Made Easy®

Third Edition

Revised by

Sachin Khanduri MD
Head
Department of Radiodiagnosis
ERA's Lucknow Medical College and Hospital
Lucknow, Uttar Pradesh, India

JAYPEE

JAYPEE BROTHERS MEDICAL PUBLISHERS
The Health Sciences Publisher
New Delhi | London

Jaypee Brothers Medical Publishers (P) Ltd.

Headquarters
EMCA House
23/23-B, Ansari Road, Daryaganj
New Delhi 110 002, India
Landline: +91-11-23272143,
+91-11-23272703
+91-11-23282021, +91-11-23245672
E-mail: jaypee@jaypeebrothers.com

Corporate Office
Jaypee Brothers Medical Publishers (P) Ltd.
4838/24, Ansari Road, Daryaganj
New Delhi 110 002, India
Phone: +91-11-43574357
Fax: +91-11-43574314
E-mail: jaypee@jaypeebrothers.com

Overseas Office
JP Medical Ltd.
83, Victoria Street, London
SW1H 0HW (UK)
Phone: +44-20 3170 8910
E-mail: info@jpmedpub.com

EU GPSR Authorised Representative
Logos Europe, 9 rue Nicolas Poussin
17000, La Rochelle, France
Phone: +33 (0) 6 67 93 73 78
E-mail: Contact@logoseurope.eu

Website: www.jaypeebrothers.com
Website: www.jaypeedigital.com

Inquiries for bulk sales may be solicited at: jaypee@jaypeebrothers.com

Karthikeyan's Chest X-ray Made Easy®

First Edition: 2007
Second Edition: 2017
Third Edition: **2025**

ISBN: 978-93-6616-273-7

Printed in India

Preface to the Third Edition

It is with great pleasure that I present the third edition of *Chest X-ray Made Easy*. Since the release of the first edition, there have been significant advancements and challenges in the field of diagnostic imaging, particularly in the interpretation of chest X-rays. The feedback from students, radiologists, and clinicians alike has been invaluable in shaping this updated edition, and we are grateful for the continued support from the medical community.

This edition builds on the foundation of the original text while incorporating important new content. In particular, we have added a dedicated chapter on *Basic Chest X-ray Findings in COVID-19*. The understanding of COVID-19's radiologic manifestations has evolved rapidly, and this chapter serves as a concise guide to recognizing the disease's patterns on chest X-rays, an essential skill during these times.

Other key updates include:

- **X-ray basics:** A comprehensive introduction to the fundamental principles of chest X-ray interpretation, designed for ease of understanding for medical students, trainees, and allied health professionals.
- **A spectrum of chest disease patterns:** This section offers an extensive account of various chest X-ray findings associated with a wide range of pulmonary conditions, from infections to malignancies.
- **Differential diagnosis of chest X-ray pathologies:** Building on the spectrum of disease patterns, this chapter equips the reader with practical tools for differential diagnosis, essential for accurate clinical decision-making.
- **Case discussions with CT thorax correlation:** Recognizing the growing role of computed tomography (CT) in the diagnostic process, this edition expands the discussion of chest X-ray cases with corresponding CT images. This correlation provides a more thorough understanding of the diseases and demonstrates how

complementary imaging modalities can enhance diagnostic accuracy.

- **Multiple choice questions (MCQs):** To enhance learning and reinforce key concepts, we have introduced MCQs at the end of each chapter. These questions will help readers test their knowledge and apply the principles they have learned in real-world scenarios, making this edition more interactive and learner-friendly.

We would also like to take this opportunity to sincerely thank the author of the first edition, whose pioneering work laid the foundation for this book. Their original contributions continue to be of immense value, and it is their vision that has guided the creation of the third edition. We are honored to build upon their legacy.

In addition, we extend our heartfelt gratitude to the postgraduate students of the department, whose invaluable assistance in writing this edition has been instrumental. Their dedication in collecting resources from various sources and helping to shape the content of this book has greatly enriched the quality of this edition. We are immensely grateful for their contributions and offer them our best wishes for their future endeavors.

The aim of this edition remains the same: To demystify chest X-ray interpretation and make it accessible for all levels of medical practitioners. Whether you are a beginner learning to navigate your first X-rays or a seasoned clinician looking for a quick reference, we hope this edition will serve as a valuable resource.

Thank you for choosing *Chest X-ray Made Easy* as your guide, and we hope you find this edition both informative and practical.

Sachin Khanduri

Preface to the First Edition

Traditionally, plain X-rays provide the earliest opportunity in many instances for diagnosing various pathologies of the chest providing a cost-effective rapid screening tool. In this era of modern cross-sectional imaging, plain radiograph is often undervalued, and the most significant limitation of the chest X-ray seems to be the lack of interest and experience among the students.

This book tries to present an easy-to-use practical approach to chest X-ray. We hope that we can rekindle the interests among medical students and various postgraduates to this simple but powerful diagnostic tool.

D Karthikeyan
Deepa Chegu

Acknowledgments

I am deeply grateful to the management of ERA's Lucknow Medical College and Hospital, Lucknow, Uttar Pradesh, for their unwavering support of my career aspirations and for creating a conducive academic environment that has allowed me to pursue these goals.

I extend my heartfelt thanks to Mr Mohsin Ali Khan, Mr Meesam Ali Khan, Dr Farzana Mahdi, and Dr Abbas Ali Mahdi for their invaluable contribution to my academic development.

I also appreciate the postgraduate residents I had the privilege of working with on this and other related projects. Their collaboration, along with the guidance and camaraderie of my fellow faculty members, has enriched my professional journey, teaching me much about both scientific research and life itself. I would like to specifically acknowledge Dr Kunal Dwari, Dr Salma Khan, Dr Tanya Bansal, Dr Aastha Agrawal, and Dr Prithvi Perumal for their contributions.

A special thank you goes to my brothers, Dr Arun Khanduri and Mr Pankaj Khanduri, for their invaluable lessons and unwavering belief in me, which have been instrumental in helping me reach this point.

Above all, I am profoundly grateful to my loving and supportive wife, Dr Shobha Khanduri, who has always been by my side, and to my two wonderful children, Satvik and Ritvik, who continue to be my greatest sources of inspiration and motivation.

I am very grateful to the whole team of M/s Jaypee Brothers Medical Publishers (P) Ltd, New Delhi, India, who helped and guided me, Shri Jitendar P Vij (Group Chairman), Mr Ankit Vij (Managing Director), Mr MS Mani (Group President), Dr Madhu Choudhary (Director–Educational Publishing), Ms Pooja Bhandari [Director–Production (Books and Journals)], Mr Ajay Kumar Sharma [Deputy General Manager (Books and Journals)], Ms Sunita Katla (Executive Assistant to Group Chairman and Publishing Manager),

Ms Samina Khan (Executive Assistant to Director–Educational Publishing), Dr Jasmeet Kaur (Development Editor), Mr Vijay Kumar Bhatia (Manager–Production), Ms Seema Dogra (Cover Visualizer), Ms Neha Verma (Graphic Designer–Cover), Mr Mithlesh Singh (Proofreader), Mr Kapil Dev Sharma (Typesetter) and Mr Rajesh Ghurkundi (Graphic Designer) and their team members, for all their support to work in this project and make it a success. Without their cooperation, I could not have completed this project.

In conclusion, I am deeply obligated by too many names not appeared here.

Contents

CHAPTER 1

Production and Properties of X-rays and Positioning

BASIC PHYSICS OF X-RAY PRODUCTION

X-rays for medical diagnostic procedures or for research purposes are produced in a standard way by accelerating electrons with a high voltage and allowing them to collide with a metal target.

Depending upon the method through which the X-rays are produced, they are given different names, although they all find the same use in diagnostic medicine.

OVERVIEW: HOW X-RAYS ARE PRODUCED (FIG. 1.1)

- A current is passed through the tungsten filament and heats it up.
- As it is heated up the increased energy enables electrons to be released from the filament through **thermionic emission.**
- The electrons are attracted towards the positively charged anode and hit the tungsten target with a maximum energy determined by the tube potential (voltage).
- As the electrons bombard the target they interact via **Bremsstrahlung and characteristic interactions** which result in the conversion of energy into heat (99%) and X-ray photons (1%).

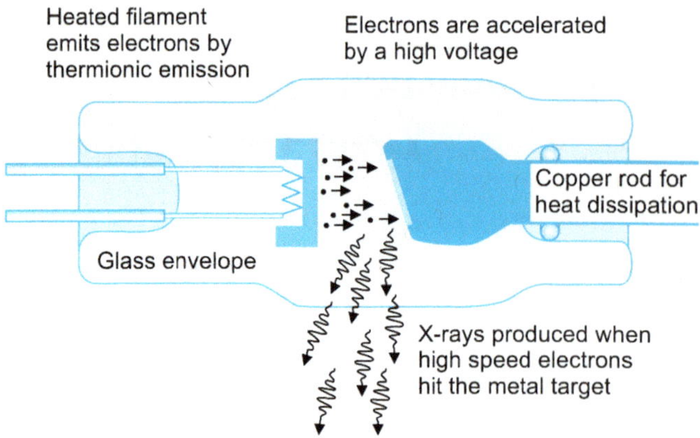

Fig. 1.1: Production of X-rays.

- The X-ray photons are released in a beam with a range of energies (**X-ray spectrum**) out of the window of the tube and form the basis for X-ray image formation.

EQUIPMENT FOR X-RAY PRODUCTION

Cathode

Filament

- Made of thin (0.2 mm) tungsten wire because tungsten:
  - Has a high atomic number (A 184, Z 74) **(Fig. 1.2)**
  - Is a good thermionic emitter (good at emitting electrons)
  - Can be manufactured into a thin wire
  - Has a very high melting temperature (3,422°C)
- The size of the filament relates to the size of the focal spot. Some cathodes have two filaments for broad and fine focusing.

Focusing Cup

- Made of molybdenum as:
  - High melting point

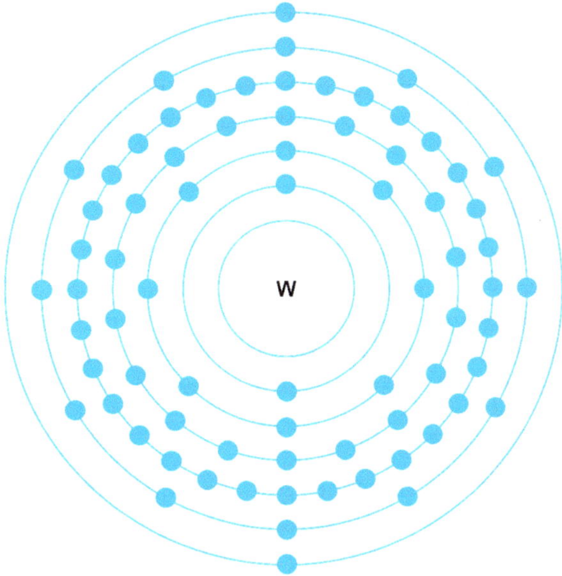

Fig. 1.2: Tungsten atom (atomic mass (A): 184, atomic number (Z): 74).

    - Poor thermionic emitter so electrons aren't released to interfere with electron beam from filament
- Negatively charged to focus the electrons towards the anode and stop spatial spreading

Anode

- Target made of tungsten for same reasons as for filament
- Rhenium added to tungsten to prevent cracking of anode at high temperatures
- Set into an anode disk of molybdenum with stem
- Positively charged to attract electrons
- Set at angle to direct X-ray photon beam down towards patient. The usual angle is 5°–15°.

Stationary Anode

These are generally limited to dental radiology and radiotherapy systems. Consists of an anode fixed in position with the electron beam constantly streaming onto one small area.

Rotating Anode

Used in most radiography, including mobile sets and fluoroscopy. Consists of a disc with a thin beveled rim of tungsten around the circumference that rotates at 50 Hz. Because it rotates it overcomes heating by having different areas exposed to the electron stream over time.

Heating of the Anode and its Removal

Heat is normally removed from the anode by **radiation** through the vacuum and into the conducting oil outside the glass envelope. The molybdenum stem conducts very little heat to prevent damage to the metal bearings.

Tube Rating

Each machine has a different capacity for dissipating heat before damage is caused. The capacity for each focal spot on a machine is given in tube rating graphs provided by the manufacturer. These display the maximum power (kV and mA) that can be used for a given exposure time before the system overloads.

Other factors to take into consideration are:

- By using a higher mA the maximum kV is reduced and vice versa.
- A very short examination may require a higher power to produce an adequate image. This must be taken into consideration as the tube may not be able to cope with that amount of heat production over such a short period of time.

Anode Cooling Chart

As well as withstanding high temperatures an anode must be able to release the heat quickly too. This ability is represented in the anode cooling chart. It shows how long it takes for the anode to cool down from its maximum level of heat and is used to prevent damage to the anode by giving sufficient time to cool between exposures.

PRODUCING AN X-RAY BEAM

Producing Electrons: Thermionic Emission

A current is applied through the cathode filament, which heats up and releases electrons via thermionic emission. The electrons are accelerated towards the positive anode by a tube voltage applied across the tube. At the anode, 99% of energy from the electrons is converted into heat and only 1% is converted into X-ray photons.

Accelerating Potential

The accelerating potential is the voltage applied across the tube to create the negative to positive gradient across the tube and accelerate the electrons across the anode. It is normally 50–150 kV for radiography, 25–40 kV for mammography and 40–110 kV for fluoroscopy.

Filament Current

The current (usually 10 A) heats up the filament to impart enough energy to the electrons to be released, i.e., it affects the **number** of electrons released.

Tube Current

This is the flow of electrons to the anode and is usually 0.5–1,000 mA.

Summary

- Filament current is applied across the tungsten cathode filament (10 A) and affects the **number** of electrons released.
- Tube current is applied across the X-ray tube from cathode to anode and affects the **energy and number** of electrons released.

X-ray Production at the Anode

The electrons hit the anode with a maximum kinetic energy of the kVp and interact with the anode by losing energy via:

- **Elastic interaction:** Rare, only happens if kVp <10 eV. Electrons interact but conserve all their energy.
- **Inelastic interaction:** Causes excitation/ionization in atoms and releases energy via electromagnetic (EM) radiation and thermal energy.

Interactions

At the anode, electrons can interact with the atoms of the anode in several ways to produce X-ray photons.

1. **Outer shell interaction:** Low energy EM released and quickly converted into heat energy.
2. **Inner shell interaction:** Produces **characteristic radiation.**
3. **Nucleus field interaction:** Also known as **Bremsstrahlung.**

1. Characteristic radiation (Fig. 1.3)

1. A bombarding electron knocks a k-shell or l-shell electron out.
2. A higher shell electron moves into the empty space.
3. This movement to a lower energy state releases energy in the form of an X-ray photon.
4. The bombarding electron continues on its path but is diverted.

It is called "characteristic" as energy of emitted electrons is dependent upon the **anode material**, not on the

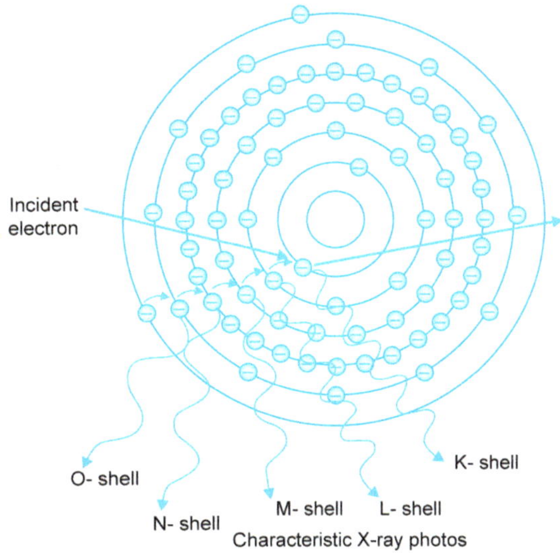

Fig. 1.3: Production of characteristic radiation.

tube **voltage**. Energy is released in characteristic values corresponding to the binding energies of different shells.

2. Bremsstrahlung radiation (Fig. 1.4)

1. Bombarding electron approaches the nucleus.
2. Electron is diverted by the electric field of the nucleus.
3. The energy loss from this diversion is released as a photon (**Bremsstrahlung radiation**).

A list of differences between **Characteristic radiation and Bremsstrahlung radiation** is summarized in **Table 1.1**.

Summary of Steps

1. **Filament current** applied through tungsten filament at cathode.

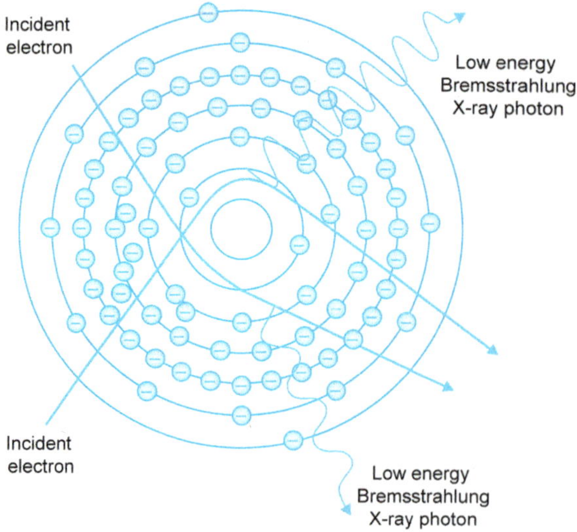

Fig. 1.4: Production of Bremsstrahlung radiation.

2. Heats up filament to produce enough energy to overcome binding energy of electrons (**thermionic emission**).
3. Electrons released from filament.
4. Tube voltage is applied across the X-ray tube.
5. Electrons, therefore, are accelerated towards positively charged anode, which gives them a certain **energy**.
6. The electrons strike the anode and the energy released via interaction with the anode atoms produces **X-ray photons**.
7. These X-ray photons leave the X-ray tube through the window in an X-ray beam towards the patient.
8. They pass through the patient to the film to produce the X-ray image.

TABLE 1.1: Differences between characteristic radiation and Bremsstrahlung radiation.

Characteristic radiation	*Bremsstrahlung radiation*
Only accounts for small percentage of X-ray photons produced	Accounts for 80% of photons in X-ray beam
Bombarding electron interacts with inner shell electron	Bombarding electron interacts with whole atom
Radiation released due to electron dropping down into lower energy state	Radiation released due to diversion of bombarding electron as a result of the atomic pull
Radiation released is of a specific energy **(Fig. 1.5)**	Radiation released is of a large range of energies **(Fig. 1.5)**
X-ray photon energy depends on element of target atoms not tube voltage	X-ray photon energy depends on tube voltage

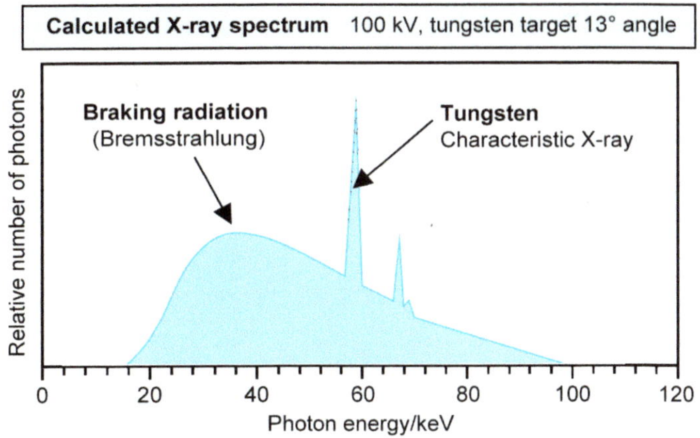

Fig. 1.5: Comparison of relative number of photons emitted with energy released in braking radiation and characteristic radiation.

COLLIMATION AND FILTRATION

A collimator is a metallic barrier (usually lead) with an aperture in the middle use to restrict size of the X-ray beam and the volume of tissue irradiated.

Collimation decreases the risk of radiation, minimizes scattered radiation, with a sharper image and better contrast.

Filtration involves removal of unwanted radiations while leaving the wanted radiation undiminished.

X-RAY SPECTRUM (FIG. 1.6)

The resulting spectrum of X-ray photon energies released is called **X-ray spectrum.** At a specific photoenergy there are peaks where more X-rays are released. These are at the **characteristic radiation** energies and are different for different materials. The rest of the graph is mainly Bremsstrahlung, in which photons with a range of energies are produced. Bremsstrahlung accounts for the majority of X-ray photon production.

Beam quality: The ability of the beam to penetrate an object or the energy of the beam.

Beam quantity: The number of X-ray photons in the beam.

The components which affects the radiographic image quality include:
- Contrast
- Dynamic range
- Spatial resolution
- Noise
- Artifacts

IMPORTANT FACTORS AFFECTING X-RAY EXPOSURE

Tube voltage (kVp), current (mAs), and **exposure time (seconds)**.

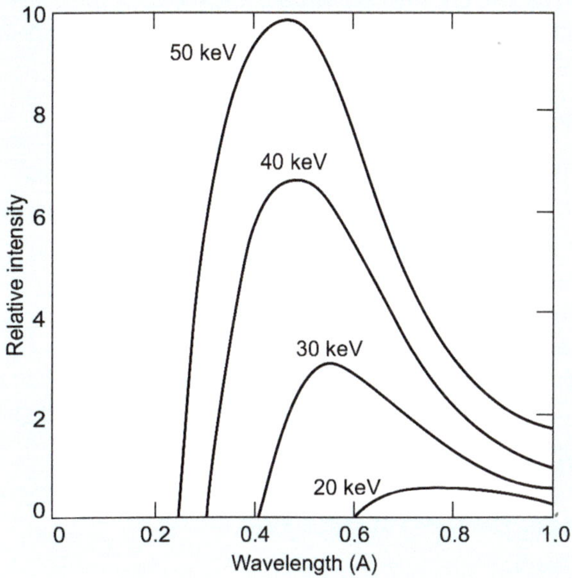

Fig. 1.6: The continuous X-ray spectrum emitted from a tungsten target four different values of e*V*, the incident electron energy.

Tube Voltage (kVp)

- The kilovoltage peak (kVp) is the difference in potential applied to the X-ray tube which is directly proportional to the average energy of the X-ray spectrum produced.
- This determines the quality of X-ray produced.
- kVp plays a role in adjusting the amount of penetration and exposure in an acquisition. An adequate penetrance ensures the ability to separate definable structures of interest; recent advances have allowed altering digital windowing levels to achieve the same effect.
- Changes in kVp affect radiation dose, exposure, and contrast.

- To achieve the best possible results, kVp is increased for sufficient exposure but kept low to minimize overexposure and radiation dose.

Current (mAs)

- Milliamperes (mA) is a unit representing the amount of current passed through the X-ray tube. Current determines the number of photons produced by the X-ray tube, also known as X-ray quantity.
- Another contributing factor toward X-ray quantity is the total exposure time, measured in seconds.
- Current and exposure time are often reported together such that: current (mA) × time (s) = milliampere-seconds (mAs).

ALTERING THE X-RAY SPECTRUM

Increasing the Tube Potential (kVp)

Increased:

- Quantity of X-ray photons
- Average energy
- Maximum energy

Increasing the Tube Current (mA)

Increased quantity of X-ray photons

No change in:

- Characteristic energy
- Average energy
- Minimum energy
- Maximum energy

QUALITY AND QUANTITY OF X-RAYS

Quality of a beam of X-rays is a measure of its penetrating power. It refers to the overall energy of the beam.

TABLE 1.2: Factors affecting x-ray beam quality and quantity.

Increase in	*Result*
Voltage (kVp)	An increase in quantity and quality
Current (mAs)	An increase in quantity and no change in quality
Added filtration	A decrease in quantity and an increase in quality

Quantity refers to the number of X-ray photons in the beam.

The various factors which influence the *quantity* and/or the *quality* of the X-ray beam (Table 1.2):

- **Quality is directly affected by,**
  i. Changes in kVp.
  ii. Changes in the atomic number (Z) of the target material.
  iii. Changes in the filtration.
  iv. The type of waveform used.
- **Quantity is affected by,**
  i. Changes in tube current (mA).
  ii. Changes in the filtration.
  iii. Changes in the atomic number of target.
  iv. Changes in kVp.
  v. Changes in type of waveform used.
  vi. Changes in distance from the tube (FFD).

PROPERTIES OF X-RAYS

- X-rays have shorter wavelength (0.1–10 nm).
- X-rays are electromagnetic radiation and travel in straight line with a velocity of light in vacuum.
- X-rays are unaffected by electric and magnetic fields.
- X-rays affect photographic film and form latent image.

- X-rays cause ionization in the medium.
- X-rays penetrate through substances that are opaque to visible light.
- X-rays can behave both as particle and wave.
- X-rays cause certain substances (calcium tungstate or rare earth phosphors) to fluoresce.
- X-rays produce excitation and ionization of the atoms and molecules of the substances through which they pass.
- X-rays interact with living tissues and can cause biological changes.

CHEST X-RAY POSITIONING

- Posteroanterior view (PA view) **(Fig. 1.7)**
- Lateral view **(Fig. 1.8)**
- Anteroposterior view (AP view) **(Fig. 1.9)**

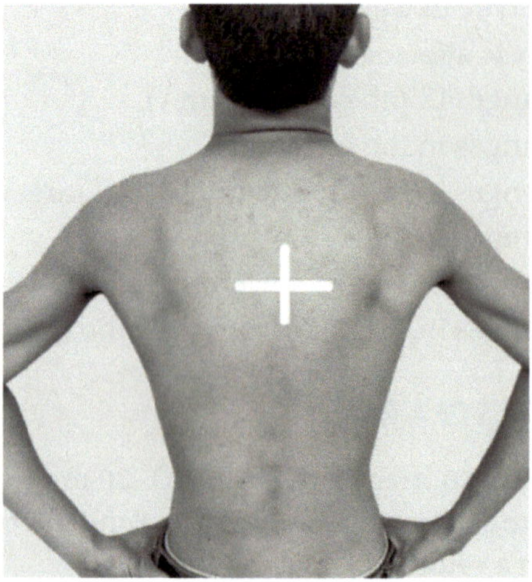

Fig. 1.7: Chest PA.

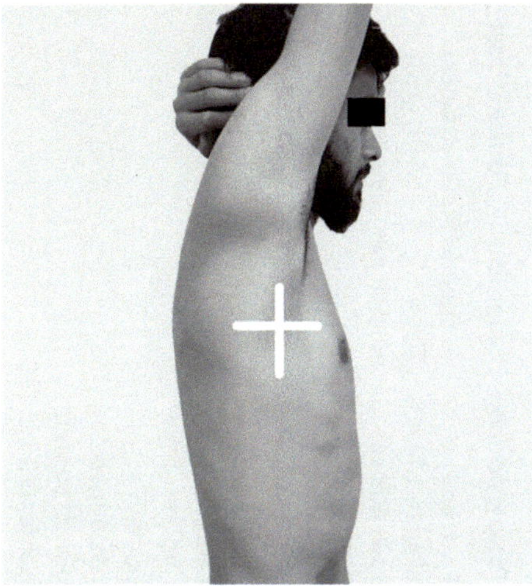

Fig. 1.8: Chest lateral.

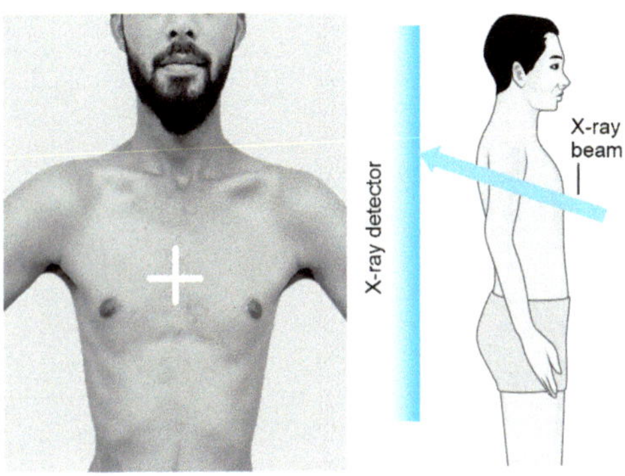

Fig. 1.9: Chest AP lordotic.

The X-ray positionings are summarized in the **Table 1.3**.

TABLE 1.3: Chest X-ray positioning.

Name	*kVp*	*Tube film distance*	*Tilt*	*Central ray*	*Patient position*	*Breathing*	*Demonstrates*
Chest PA **(Fig. 1.7)**	110 (100 to 120)	72 inches	–	To the film	PA, chin elevated, hands splaced over buttocks, and shoulders rolled forward. Thoracic spine centered to the midline of the bucky. Cassette positioned so that its superior border is 2 inches above the shoulders	Suspended deep inspiration	Lung fields, heart, great vessels, ribs, shoulder girdles, thoracic spine and upper abdomen

Contd...

Contd...

Name	*kVp*	*Tube film distance*	*Tilt*	*Central ray*	*Patient position*	*Breathing*	*Demonstrates*
Chest LAT **(Fig. 1.8)**	110 (100 to 120)	72 inches	–	To the film	Left lateral position, with no rotation. Both arms elevated and crossed on top of the head. Cassette position is 2 inches above the shoulders	Suspended deep inspiration	Lung fields, heart, great vessels, ribs, sternum and thoracic spine
Chest AP lordotic **(Fig. 1.9)**	110 (100 to 120)	66 inches	30° caudally	To the film	Upright AP patient tilt: Patient stands 1 foot from the bucky and leans back, with shoulders, neck, and back of the head against bucky	Suspended full inspiration	Lung apices, right middle lobe and lingular segments

MULTIPLE CHOICE QUESTIONS

1. Contrast in X-ray is dependent on:
   a. KV
   b. mA
   c. Duration of exposure
   d. Distance between source and object

2. X-ray films are least sensitive to which light:
   a. Violet
   b. Blue
   c. Yellow
   d. Red

3. Speed of X-ray is equal to:
   a. Speed of light
   b. Speed of electron in X-ray tube
   c. Tube voltage
   d. All of the above

4. X-rays are formed when electron hits:
   a. Anode
   b. Radium source
   c. Copper
   d. None of the above

5. Target material which produces X-rays in a diagnostic X-ray tube is made up of:
   a. Lead
   b. Tungsten
   c. Cobalt
   d. Copper

6. 1 Gray of radiation is equal to:
   a. 1 Rad
   b. 10 Rad
   c. 100 Rad
   d. 1,000 Rad

7. X-rays are produced by:
   a. Electron
   b. Neutron
   c. Protons
   d. Positrons

8. Thickness of lead in lead apron is:
   a. 5 mm
   b. 0.5 mm
   c. 0.5 cm
   d. 50 mm

9. Atomic number of Tungsten:

a. 72
b. 74
c. 76
d. 78

10. The photoelectric interaction occurs primarily in:

a. L-shell
b. K-shell
c. Outer shell
d. All shells equally

11. Electromagnetic wave has:

a. High energy high frequency
b. High energy low frequency
c. Low energy high frequency
d. Low energy low frequency

12. In a modern rotatory anode X-ray tube cooling is done by:

a. Convection
b. Conduction
c. Radiation
d. None of the above

ANSWERS

1. a
2. d
3. a
4. a
5. b
6. c
7. a
8. b
9. b
10. b
11. a
12. c

CHAPTER 2

Chest X-ray

INTRODUCTION

Radiology is an indispensable part of clinical medicine. The chest X-ray is the most commonly performed radiographic examination. It is usually recommended as the initial investigation for patients with complaints of shortness of breath, persistent cough, chest pain or a chest injury.

The ability to evaluate and understand this aspect of conventional radiology is critical for medical students entering their clinical years and for physicians throughout their careers.

OBJECTIVES OF CHEST X-RAY

1. Identify normal cardiothoracic anatomical structures demonstrable on a chest film.
2. Recognize radiographic signs of lung pathologies like atelectasis, consolidation, pneumothorax, pleural and pericardial effusions, hyperinflation, etc.
3. Correlate physical signs and symptoms of cardiopulmonary disease with chest radiographic findings.

STANDARD VIEWS

- Posteroanterior (PA)
- Lateral X-ray
- Anteroposterior (AP).

SPECIAL VIEWS

The frontal and lateral projections suffice for most radiographic purposes. Other special views include:

- Lordotic view
- Inspiration and expiration film
- Reverse lordotic view
- Oblique
- Supine (bedside CXR)
- Lateral decubitus film.

High Penetration Film with Moving Grid (Bucky Film)

1. Obesity
2. Dense pleural or pulmonary opacities
3. Calcified lesions
4. Lesions obscured by heart or diaphragms
5. Air bronchograms in densely infiltrated areas.

To show the hidden areas on PA view (mediastinum, hila), rib destruction, cavitation, calcification, airways; a penetrated film should be obtained.

Intrathoracic Pressure Maneuvers

1. **Valsalva maneuver:** Shrinks pulmonary vessels
2. **Muller maneuver:** Distends pulmonary vessels.

Indications

a. Distinguish blood vessel from lymph node
b. Distinguish A-V malformation from solid lesion.

Supine Film

a. *Decreases lung volume*—highlights infiltrates and interstitium.
b. *Increases venous return to heart*—distends azygos vein and pulmonary vein.

c. *Diaphragm rises and intracardiac pressure increases*—heart and mediastinal structures enlarge.
- Fluid and air migrate.
- Pleural effusions disappear.
- Small pneumothorax disappears.
- Air-fluid levels (e.g., lung abscess) disappear.

Pneumothorax Signs on Supine Film

1. Deep sulcus sign
   a. Costophrenic angle sharply outlined by air
   b. Diaphragm-mediastinal junction sharply outlined
2. Hyperlucency superimposed over liver shadow.

TECHNIQUES

The ideal radiograph provides image of structures within the chest using minimum radiation.

PA View

The standard chest examination consists of a PA (posterior-anterior) and lateral chest X-ray.
- The patient should be examined in full inspiration.
- Patient's chest is placed against the cassette.
- The PA view minimizes cardiac magnification which can complicate other views.

Lateral View

A lateral view is ordered in conjunction with a PA view.

Left side of the chest is conventionally placed against the cassette.

Since the right side of the body is closer to the source of the X-rays, the right side is magnified greater than the left side.

This view may expose lesions that are retrosternal or hidden by the diaphragm. The patient is placed with the film against the side of the chest where the lesion is suspected. For example, a left lateral view (with the left side of the chest held against the film) would be used to examine the area behind the left side of the heart. It is best when the lesion is as close to the film as possible.

AP View

It is performed on patients who are unable to stand for the PA exam.

- Performed at the bedside.
- This view may cause cardiac magnification.

AP view is sometimes useful to determine whether a questionable opacity on PA view is genuine by altering the position of overlying ribs. AP view also provides better visualization of posterior chest.

Lordotic View

Useful to demonstrate lung apices free from superimposed shadows of clavicle and first rib and middle lobe pathologies like middle lobe collapse/consolidation.

Lateral Decubitus (Fig. 2.1)

Helpful to assess the volume of pleural effusion and demonstrate whether a pleural effusion is mobile or loculated. It is a sensitive method for detecting small quantities of pleural fluid (50–100 mL) and also to differentiate between subpulmonic effusion and high diaphragm. Also helps to assess the nondependent hemithorax to confirm a pneumothorax in a patient who could not be examined erect. Additionally, the dependent lung should increase in density due to atelectasis from the weight of the mediastinum putting pressure on it. Failure to do so indicates air trapping.

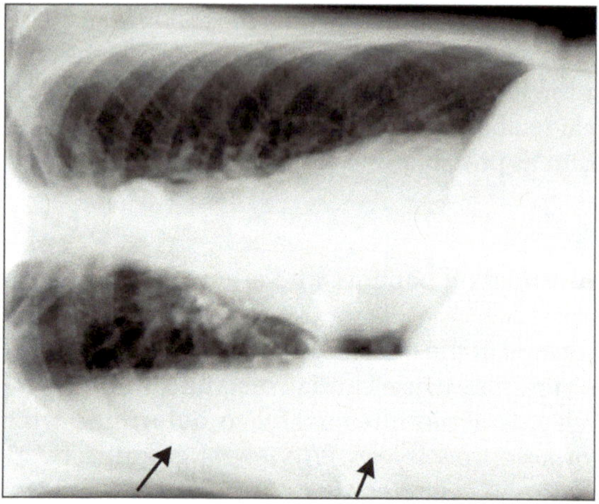

Fig. 2.1: Lateral decubitus X-ray.

Paired Inspiratory-Expiratory View

Films exposed in expiration is important in the investigation of air trapping, e.g., in cases of foreign body aspiration. An expiratory film is also helpful to demonstrate small pneumothorax. Diaphragmatic function is also well-assessed on expiratory films.

Oblique View

Useful to demonstrate pleural plaques, chest wall lesions, rib lesions and lower lobe collapse.

TECHNICAL CONSIDERATIONS

Inspiration (Fig. 2.2)

The patient should be examined in full inspiration. This greatly helps the radiologist to determine if there are intrapulmonary abnormalities. The diaphragm should be found at about the level of the 8th–10th posterior rib or 5th–6th anterior rib on good inspiration.

Penetration (Figs. 2.3, 2.4 and Table 2.1)

Adequate penetration of the patient by radiation is also required for a good film. On a good PA film, the thoracic spine disc spaces should be barely visible through the heart but bony details of the spine are not usually seen. On the other hand penetration is sufficient that bronchovascular structures can usually be seen through the heart.

On the lateral view, you can look for proper penetration and inspiration by observing that the spine appears to darken as you move caudally. This is due to more air in lung in the lower lobes and less chest wall. The sternum should be seen edge on and posteriorly you should see two sets of ribs.

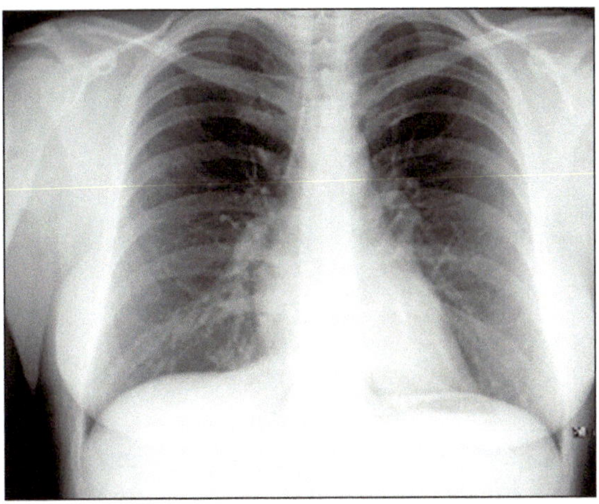

Fig. 2.2: PA view in good inspiration.

Rotation (Figs. 2.5 to 2.7)

The technologists are usually very careful to X-ray the patient flat against the cassette. If there is rotation of the patient, the mediastinum may look very unusual. One can access patient rotation by observing the clavicular heads and determining whether they are in equal distance from the spinous process of the thoracic vertebral bodies.

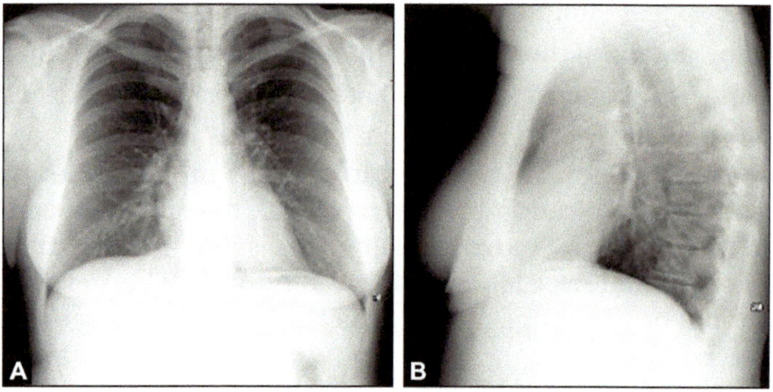

Figs. 2.3A and B: Normal PA and lateral chest X-ray.

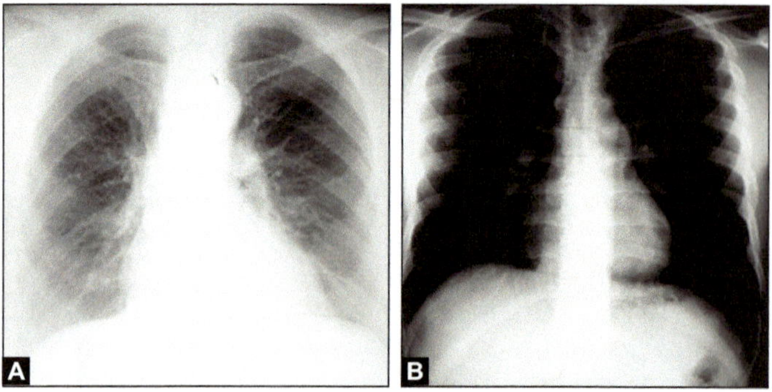

Figs. 2.4A and B: (A) Underpenetrated radiograph; (B) Overpenetrated radiograph.

TABLE 2.1: Penetration factor: Underpenetrated image vs overpenetrated image.

Underpenetrated	*Overpenetrated*
» Underpenetrated X-ray will emphasize normal lung and make it appear as if there are infiltrates » Left hemidiaphragm and left lung base not visible adequately » Underpenetrated chest » X-ray does not differentiate the vertebral bodies from the intervertebral spaces	» Lung fields are "blacker" than usual » There is no adequate lung detail » Absence of peripheral vasculature » See vertebrae extending down into the abdominal region

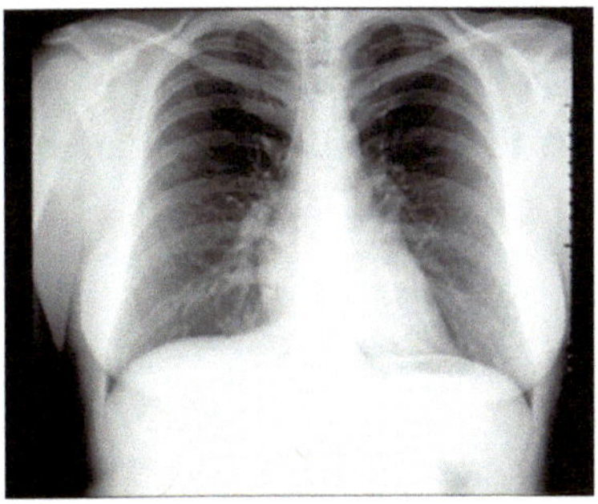

Fig. 2.5: Normal PA film without any rotation.

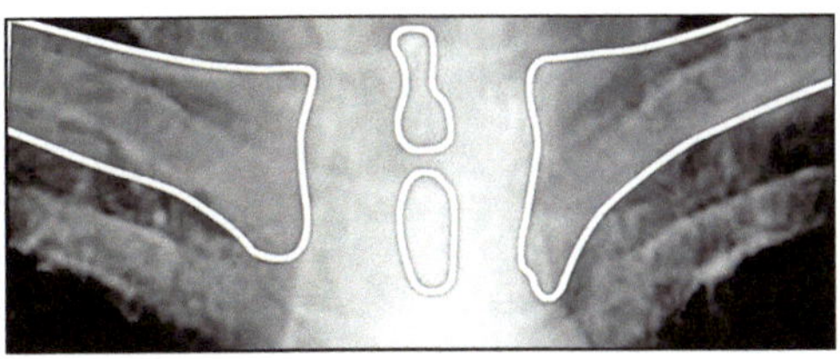

Fig. 2.6: Clavicular head and spinous process alignment showing a straight film.

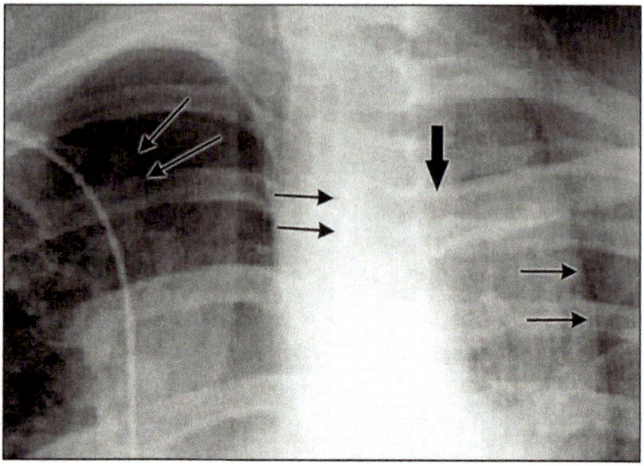

Fig. 2.7: Rotated film. Note the positioning of the heads of the clavicles (black arrows) and the spinous processes (black arrow on right). Incidental pneumothorax seen on the left (black arrows).

Normal Anatomy of Chest X-ray

Figure 2.8 shows the anatomical landmarks on a chest x-ray PA view.

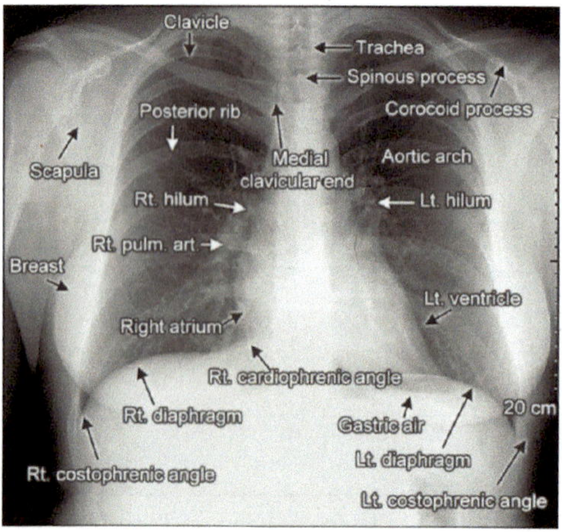

Fig. 2.8: Normal structures.

LUNG ZONES

Bronchopulmonary Segments

Each bronchial division and its accompanying pulmonary arterial branch supply a particular region of lung. This entire unit of lung is called bronchopulmonary segment. Each segment is pyramidal shaped with apex towards hilum. They are functional independent respiratory units.

Right lung has two fissures (minor and major) dividing the lung into 3 lobes—upper, middle and lower **(Table 2.2, Figs. 2.9 and 2.10)**.

TABLE 2.2: Bronchopulmonary segments in right lung (10 segments).

Upper lobe	*Middle lobe*	*Lower lobe*
» Apical	» Medial	» Apical
» Anterior	» Lateral	» Anterior basal
» Posterior		» Posterior basal
		» Medial basal
		» Lateral basal

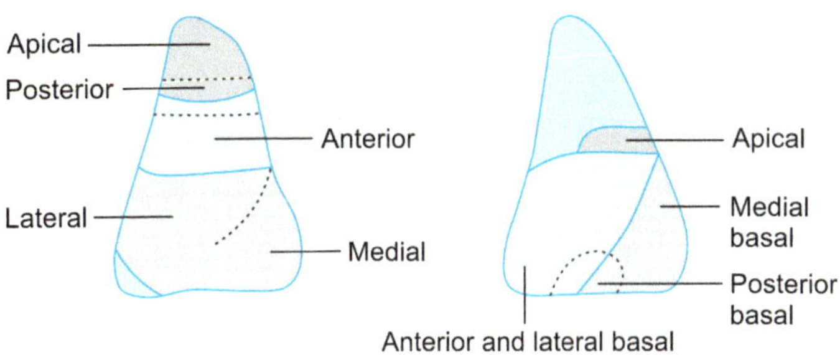

Fig. 2.9: Posteroanterior view of right lung.

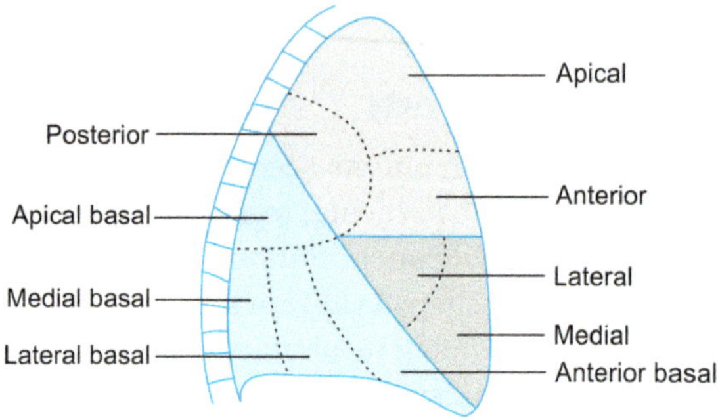

Fig. 2.10: Lateral view of right lung.

Left lung has 1 fissure (major) dividing the lung into 2 lobes—upper (includes lingual) and lower **(Table 2.3, Figs. 2.11 and 2.12)**.

TABLE 2.3: Bronchopulmonary segments in left lung (8 segments).

Upper lobe	*Lingula*	*Lower lobe*
» Apicoposterior	» Superior	» Apical
» Anterior	» Inferior	» Anteromedial basal
		» Lateral basal
		» Posterior basal

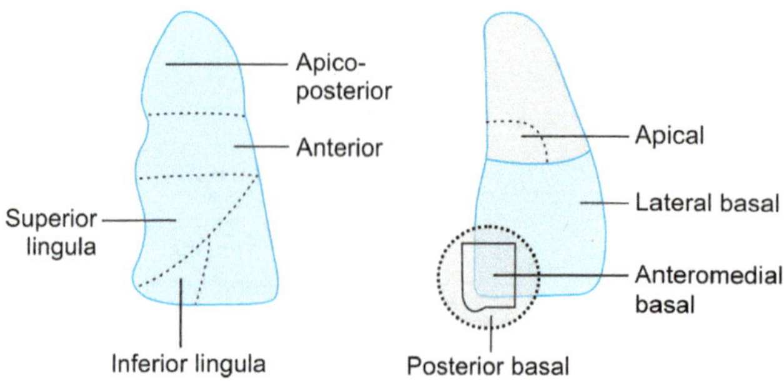

Fig. 2.11: Posteroanterior view of left lung.

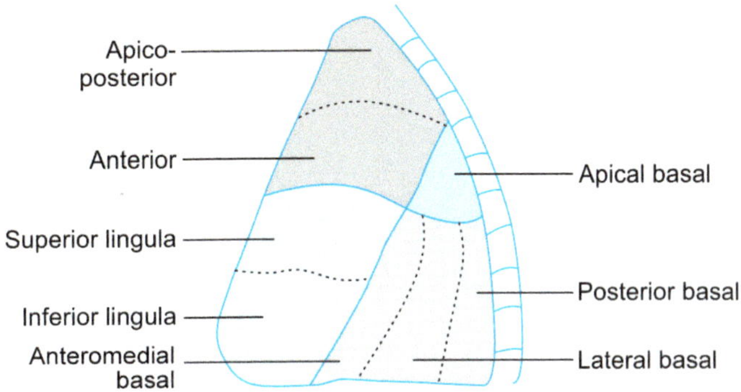

Fig. 2.12: Lateral view of left lung.

Extent of Lobes on Normal Films (Figs. 2.13 and 2.14)

These diagrams show the extent of the lobes in a normal subject, as seen on the PA and lateral films.

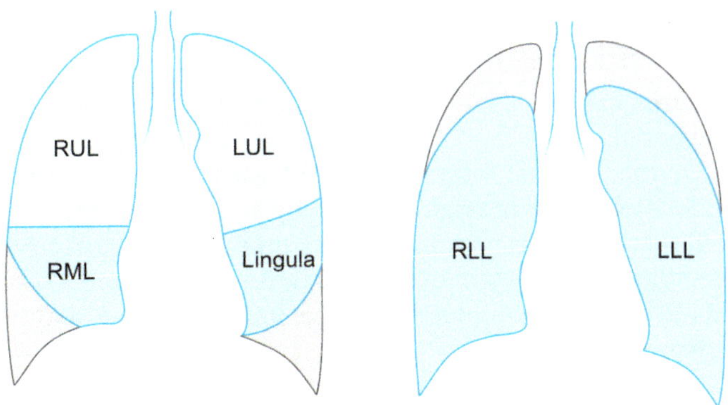

Fig. 2.13: PA view: Extent of upper and lower lobes. Note the extensive overlap. The lower lobes extend considerably higher than many realize.

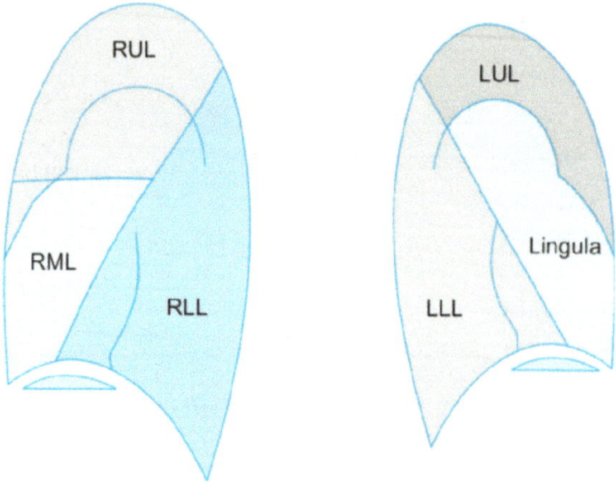

Fig. 2.14: Lateral view: Extent of lobes on the lateral view (note that the left and right sides are in practice superimposed upon one another).

FISSURES (FIGS. 2.15, 2.16 AND TABLE 2.4)

Fissures can be visualized only when the X-ray beam is tangential.

On the PA chest X-ray, the minor fissure divides the right middle lobe from the right upper lobe and is sometimes not well seen. There is no minor fissure on the left. It runs from the hilum to the region of sixth rib in the axillary line. Often this fissure is incomplete and runs anteriorly and slightly downwards.

The major fissures are usually not well seen on the PA view because you are looking through them obliquely. If there is fluid in the fissure, it is occasionally manifested as a density at the lower lateral margin. Both major fissures start posteriorly at the level T4/T5 and passes through the hilum. The left is steeper and ends 5 cm behind the anterior costophrenic angle and the right major fissure ends just behind the costophrenic angle.

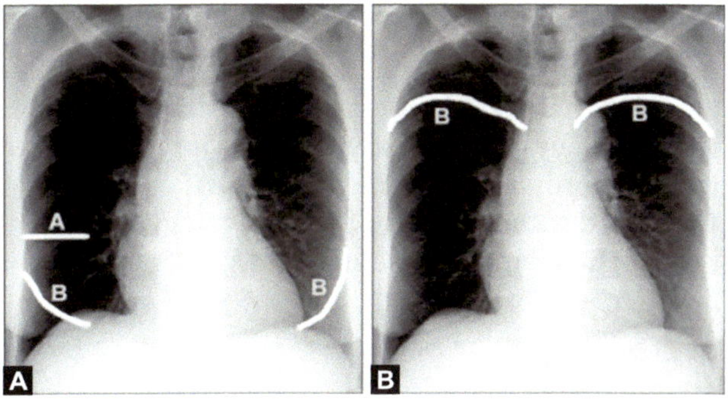

Figs. 2.15A and B: Right minor fissure (A) Superior and inferior border of the major. Inferior fissures; (B) Bilaterally.

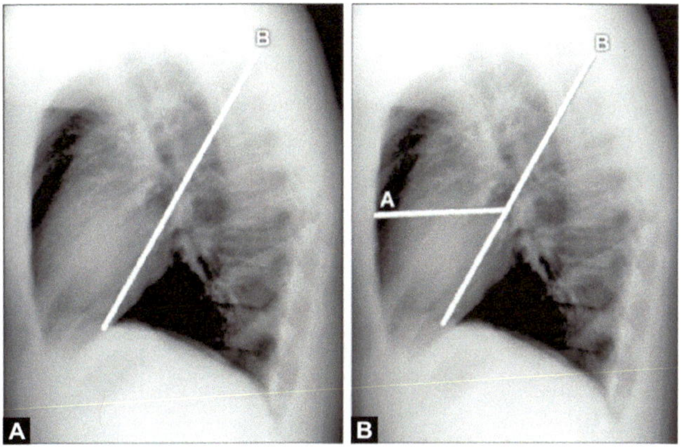

Figs. 2.16A and B: On the lateral view, both lungs are superimposed. The left lung has only a major fissure (B). The right lung will have both the major (B) and minor fissure (A).

TABLE 2.4: Major fissures of lungs.	
Left major oblique fissure	Separates the LUL from the LLL
Right major fissure	Separates the RUL/RML from the RLL
Right minor fissure	Separates the RUL from the RML

Accessory Fissures

1. **Azygos fissure:** Comma shaped. Usually seen in the apex of right lung. It contains paired folds of parietal and visceral pleura with the azygos vein which has failed to migrate normally **(Figs. 2.17 and 2.18)**.
2. **Left-sided minor fissure:** Separates lingual from other upper lobe segments.

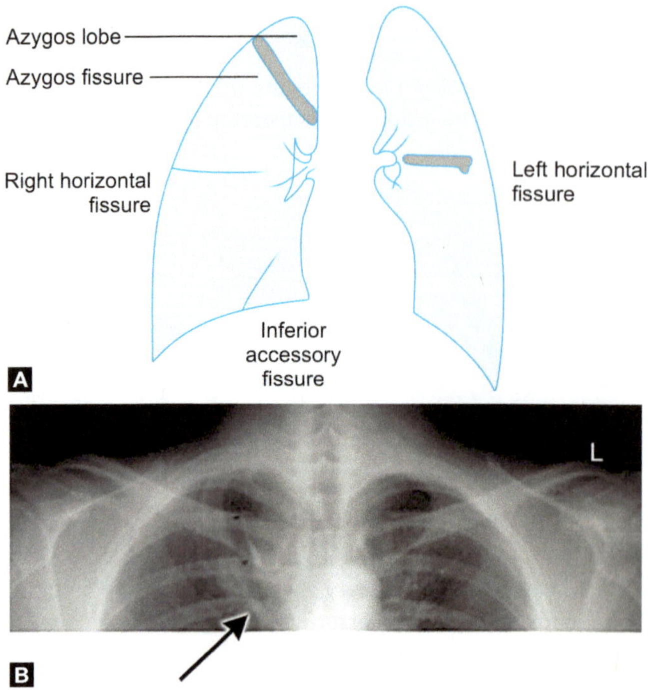

Figs. 2.17A and B: (A) Schematic of chest AP view showing azygous fissure; (B) Chest X-ray showing azygos fissure.

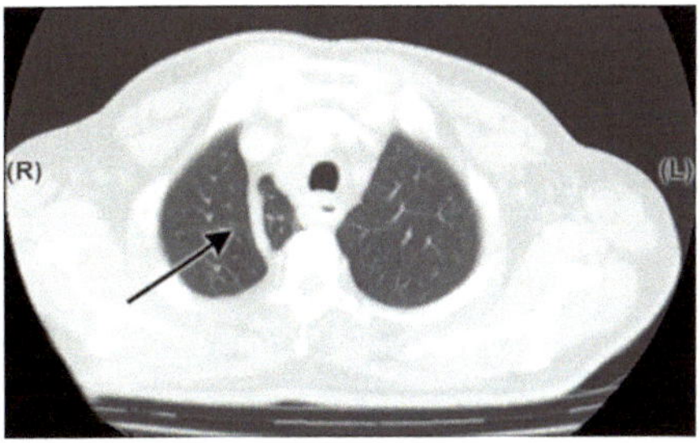

Fig. 2.18: Axial CT of lung showing the azygos fissure.

3. **Superior accessory fissure:** Common on right side (in 5% of population). On PA view it resembles minor fissure and separates apical from basal segments of lower lobe. On lateral view this fissure is seen to run posteriorly from the hilum **(Figs. 2.19A and B)**.

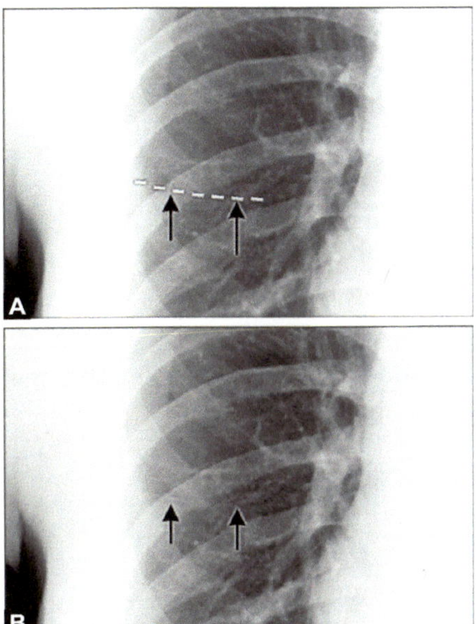

Figs. 2.19A and B: CXR showing the course of the superior accessory fissure.

4. **Inferior accessory fissure:** Common on the right side and runs up from cardiophrenic angle obliquely. Usually separates medial basal segment from the rest of the basal segments **(Figs. 2.20A and B)**.

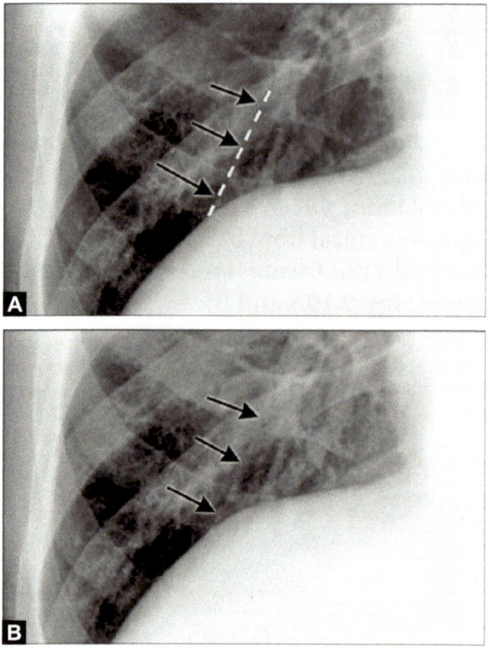

Figs. 2.20A and B: CXR showing the course of the inferior accessory fissure.

MEDIASTINUM AND HEART

Mediastinum (Figs. 2.23, 2.26 and 2.27)

Mediastinum separates the thoracic cavity into right and left pleural spaces. It extends from thoracic inlet to the diaphragm and is enveloped by parietal pleura. It extends anteriorly to the sternum and posteriorly to paravertebral gutters.

Central dense shadow on PA view consists of mediastinum and spine sternum.

Division of Mediastinum

Conventional Method (Figs. 2.21)

Mediastinum is conventionally divided into superior, anterior, middle and posterior compartments.

- **Superior mediastinum:** Extends from thoracic inlet superiorly to an imaginary line joining sternal angle and 4th intervertebral disk space inferiorly.
- **Anterior mediastinum:** Space bounded by sternum anteriorly and posteriorly by pericardium.
- **Middle mediastinum:** Space containing pericardium and contents, trachea, vena cava.
- **Posterior mediastinum:** Space posterior to pericardium upto paravertebral gutters.

Felson's Method (Fig. 2.22)

In this method, anterior mediastinum includes the space anterior to the line drawn along the posterior margin of pericardium and anterior to the trachea. This space includes the heart.

Middle mediastinum includes trachea and all structures anterior to a line drawn 1 cm posterior to the anterior border of vertebral body.

Posterior mediastinum includes paravertebral gutters.

Other methods: Sutton's method, Heitzman's method.

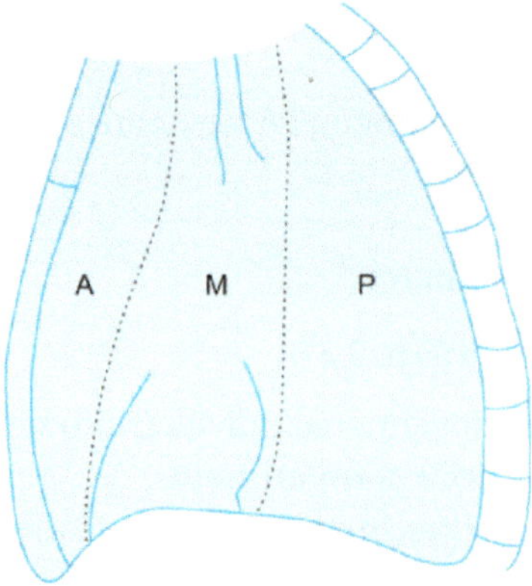

Fig. 2.21: Schematic diagram showing the anatomical division of mediastinum (A = anterior; M = middle; P = posterior).

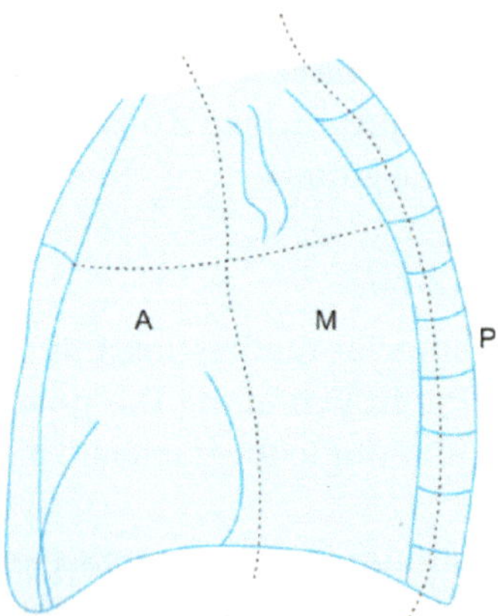

Fig. 2.22: Schematic diagram of Felsons mediastinal divisions (A = anterior mediastinum; M = middle mediastinum; P = posterior mediastinum)

Heart (Figs. 2.23 and 2.24)

- Two-thirds of the heart lies on the left side of the chest, with one-third on the right. The heart should take up no more than half of the thoracic cavity.

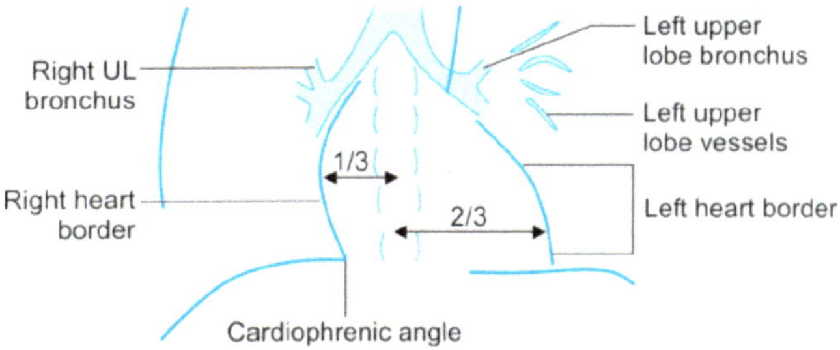

Fig. 2.23: Schematic of cardiac borders.

- The left border of the heart is made up by the left atrium and left ventricle.
- The right border is made up by the right atrium alone. Above the right heart border lies the edge of the superior vena cava. The right ventricle sits anteriorly and therefore does not have a border on the PA chest X-ray film.

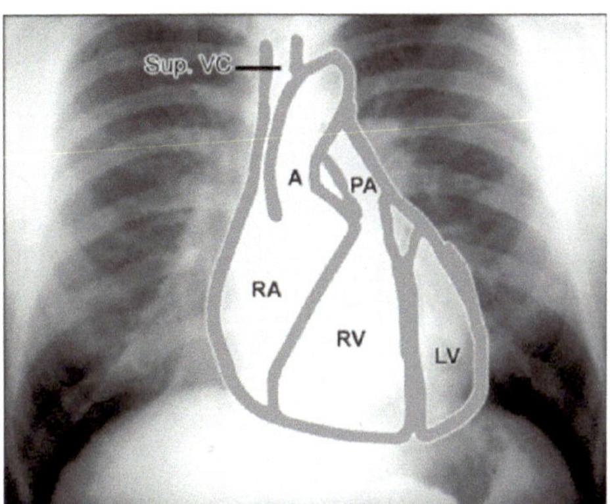

Fig. 2.24: Posteroanterior view.

- On a lateral chest X-ray, the heart lies anteroinferiorly **(Fig. 2.25)**.
- Apparent cardiac enlargement occurs with short Film-focus distance (FFD), on expiration, in AP and supine views.

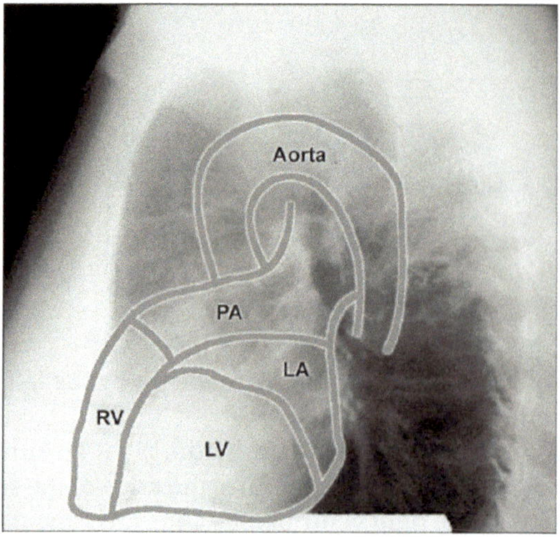

Fig. 2.25: Lateral view.

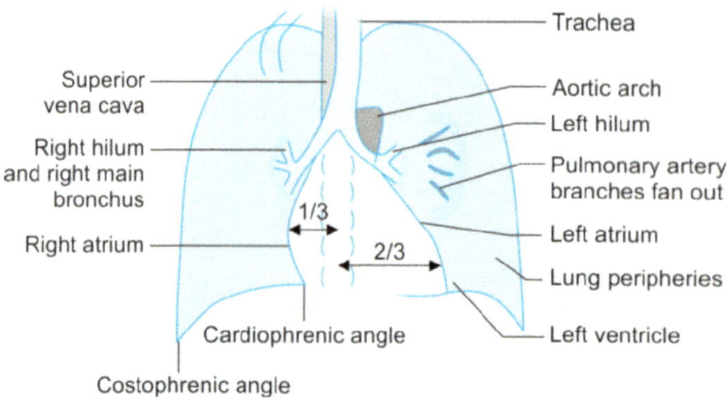

Fig. 2.26: Structures forming the mediastinal margins.

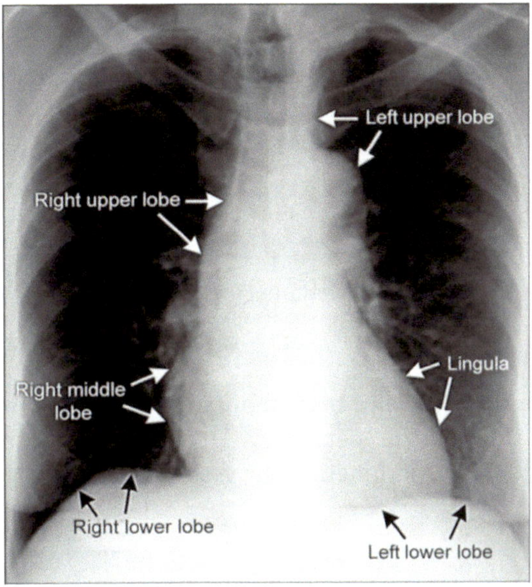

Fig. 2.27: The lobes of the lungs forming the margins of the lungs along the mediastinum and chest wall.

HILA

The "hilum" is composed of the pulmonary artery and its branches, and adjacent airway and pulmonary veins. Since airways do not produce a significant shadow on plain film radiography, the majority of the detectable "hilar" structures are vascular.

The pulmonary arteries and upper lobe veins significantly contribute to the hilar shadow on plain chest X-ray.

Left hilum is slightly at a higher position (0.5–2 cm) than the right hilum. Both the hila should be of equal size, density with concave lateral borders. Normal lymph nodes are not seen.

The right pulmonary artery courses below the level of left main stem bronchus. As a result, the right hilar shadow is inferior to the left on the PA projection. This is seen in 70% of the population. In the rest of the 30%, the hilar shadows are equal in height.

The right pulmonary artery is approximately 3 times larger than the LPA.

On the lateral projection, the right hilum is anterior to a line drawn through the tracheal air column.

Pulmonary Vessels (Figs. 2.28 and 2.29)

The arteries and veins branch out from the hila, becoming smaller towards the periphery. The larger central vessels are better seen; peripherally the vessels overlap as they run laterally.

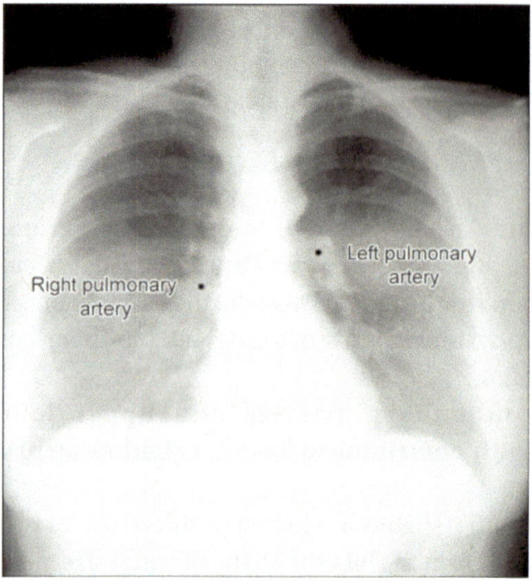

Fig. 2.28: Pulmonary arteries.

In the upright position, the lower lung vessels are larger than the upper lung vessels, due to gravitational effects on flow. If the patient is supine, there is redistribution (increase) in flow to the upper lung vessels. This is called cephalization of flow. Congestive heart failure also causes redistribution to the upper lung vessels, even when the patient is upright when the X-ray film is taken.

On the left side, the left pulmonary artery is directed posterolaterally, towards the left scapula. This artery goes over the left main stem bronchus, and therefore, the left pulmonary artery is located higher than the right pulmonary artery. On the lateral projection, the left pulmonary artery is posterior to a line drawn down the tracheal air column.

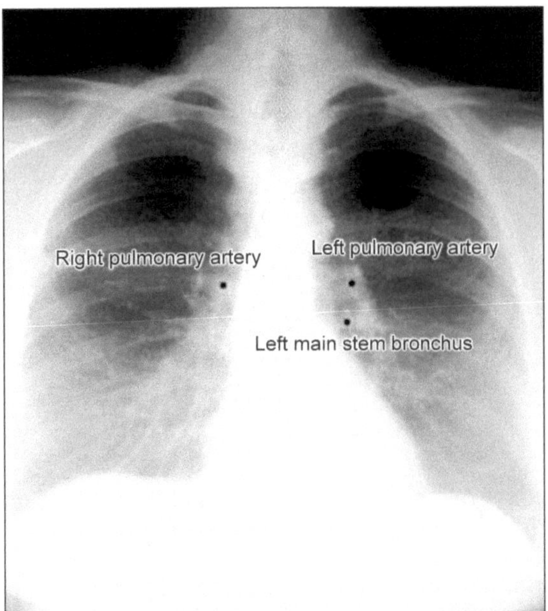

Fig. 2.29: Relationship of artery and bronchus.

DIAPHRAGM

Diaphragm is a dome-shaped musculotendinous partition that separates thoracic cavity from abdominal cavity. It is formed by fusion of septum transversum, dorsal mesogastrium, pleuroperitoneal folds and side wall mesenchyme.

It has sternal, costal and vertebral origin.

It consists of a central tendon, with right and left leaflets composed of striated muscles. Three large openings disrupt the continuity of the diaphragm: the aortic, esophageal, and inferior vena caval apertures. The diaphragm is covered by parietal pleura and peritoneum except for the bare area ofthe liver. Anatomically, the diaphragm is composed of two parts: the lumbar diaphragm and costal diaphragm.

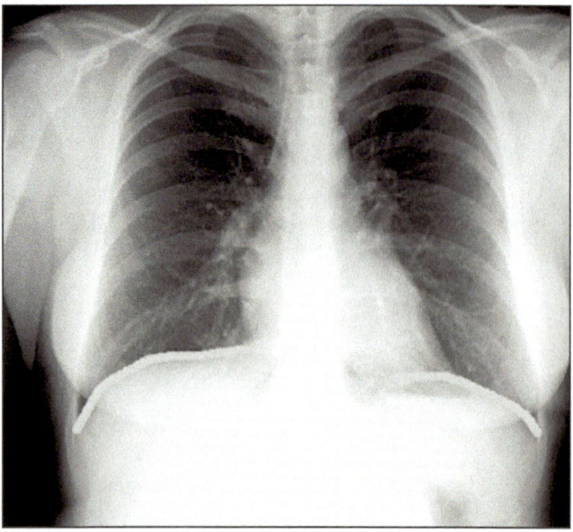

Fig. 2.30: Right dome higher than the left dome.

Diaphragm has smooth outline in most individuals. Angle of contact with the chest wall is acute and sharp. Blunting of the angle is sometimes normally seen in athletes. Normally right hemidiaphragm is 1.5–2.5 cm higher than the left and is usually at the level of 6th rib anteriorly **(Fig. 2.30)**. Difference of more than 3 cm is considered abnormal. In 3% of population, left hemidiaphragm is at a higher level than the right.

Normal excursion of the diaphragm is between 1.5 and 2.5 cm.

Check for flattening of dome of diaphragm by drawing a line perpendicular from the midpoint of the dome to a line joining costophrenic and cardiophrenic angles. This distance is usually >1.5 cm if it is less than 1.5 cm, then it is considered flattened **(Fig. 2.31)**.

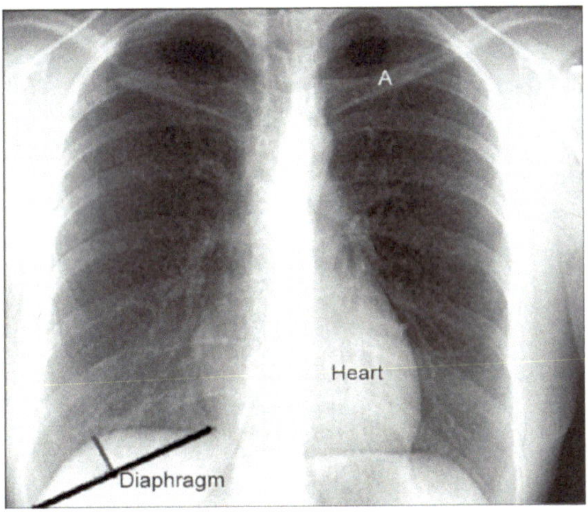

Fig. 2.31: CXR showing the method of measuring the dome.

Check for the presence of the gastric gas bubble below the left hemidiaphragm **(Figs. 2.32A and B)**.

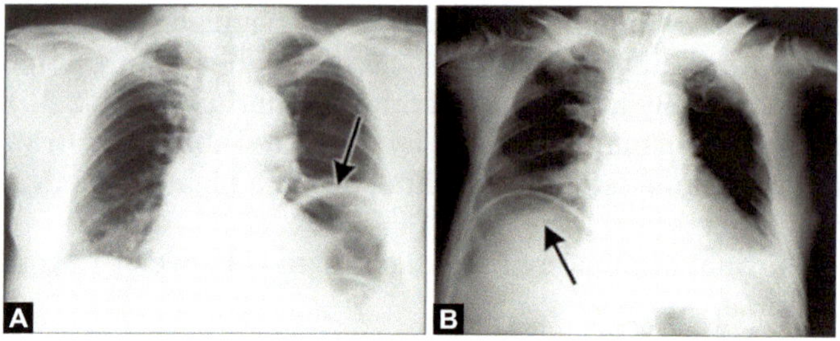

Figs. 2.32A and B: (A) Normal; (B) Large gastric bubble.

Look below the diaphragm for any evidence of free air **(Figs. 2.33A and B)**.

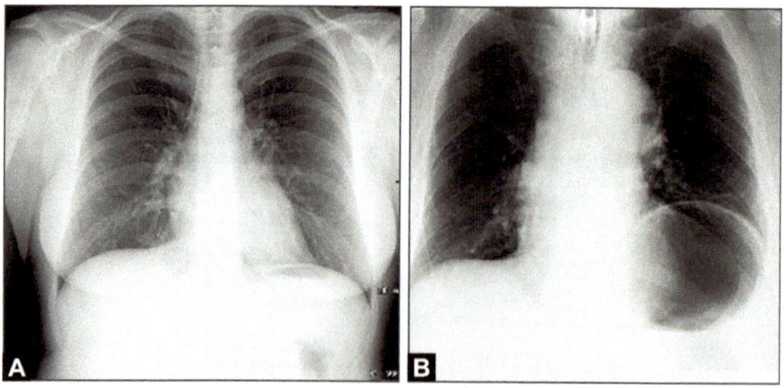

Figs. 2.33A and B: (A) Eventration of left hemidiaphragm; (B) Air under the diaphragm.

Normal Variants (Fig. 2.34)

1. Scalloping
2. Muscle slips
3. Diaphragmatic humps and dromedary diaphragm
4. Eventration
5. Accessory diaphragm

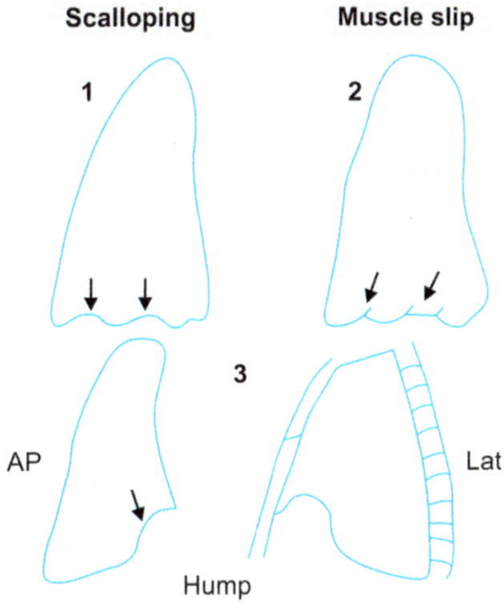

Fig. 2.34: Diaphragmatic contours.

INTERPRETATION: *How to look at a Chest PA view*

COMPARISON WITH PREVIOUS X-RAYS

This is often the single most important diagnostic maneuver in the interpretation of chest roentgenograms. Every effort should be made to obtain previous films for comparison with the current films.

The easiest way to identify a new abnormality is to note its absence on a previous film!!

The key to successfully interpreting any radiograph is to be systematic.

Examine all parts of the film in an orderly manner, and do this consistently.

Identification

1. Correct patient
2. Correct date and time
3. Correct examination

Side Marker

The position of side marker allows the radiograph to be oriented correctly for reading.

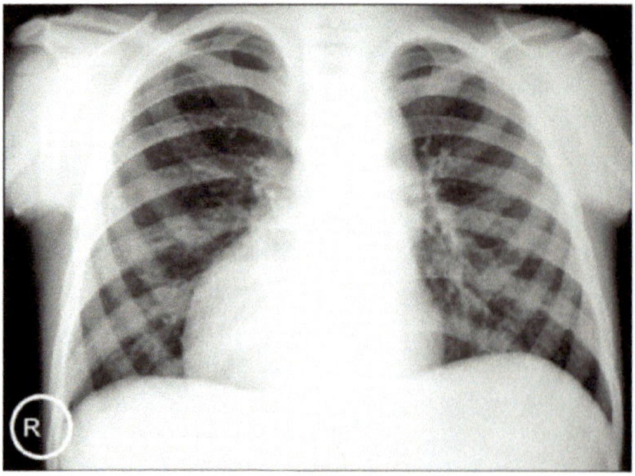

Fig. 2.35: Note the dextrocardia, easily noted if the side marker is placed correctly.

Technique

Next concentrate on the technical factors:

1. Is the examination complete?
2. Are all the requested views included?
3. Is the entire anatomical area included on the films?
   a. Projection
   b. Position
   c. Penetration
   d. Rotation
   e. Inspiration.

Systematic Analysis

1. Soft tissue including breast, chest wall, companion shadow.
2. Bones—shoulder girdles, spine and rib cage.

3. Diaphragm position, shape, subdiaphragmatic abnormalities.
4. Review abdomen for bowel gas, organ size, abnormal calcifications, free air.
5. Plastic—endotracheal tube, lines, tubes.
6. **Review mediastinum:**
   a. Overall size and shape.
   b. *Trachea:* Position, carina. The trachea should be central
   c. *Margins:* SVC, ascending aorta, right atrium, left subclavian artery, aortic arch, main pulmonary artery, left ventricle.
   d. *Lines and stripes:* Paratracheal, paraspinal, paraesophageal (azygoesophageal), para-aortic
   e. Retrosternal clear space.
7. **Heart size and shape:** The width of the heart should be no greater than 50% of the width of the rib cage.
8. **Review hila:**
   a. Normal relationships
   b. Size
9. **Parenchyma:** Mentally divide the entire chest into upper, middle and lower thirds. Then, methodically compare the right and left sides of each lung section looking for asymmetry. The easiest way to identify an abnormality is to confirm that it does not exist on the other side.

   Compare lung sizes, aeration, vascular distinctness, and abnormal opacities.
10. **Pleura:** Costophrenic and cardiophrenic angles, thickening fissures—major and minor—if seen.

Hidden Areas (Figs. 2.36A to C)

- Supraclavicular regions
- Ends of ribs

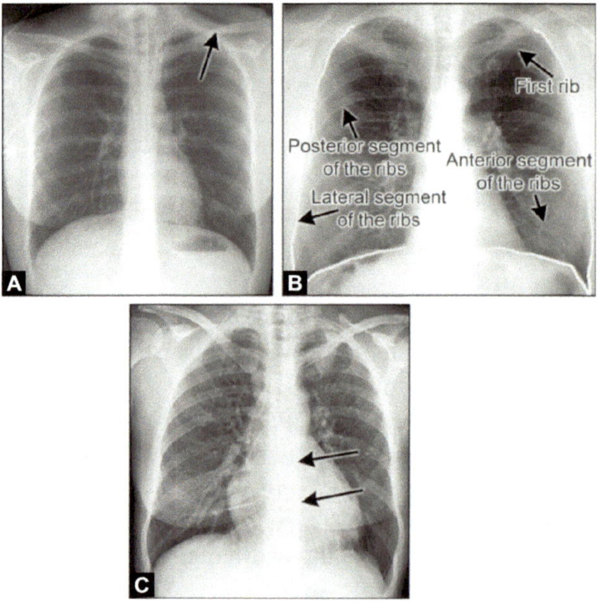

Figs. 2.36A to C: Hidden areas.

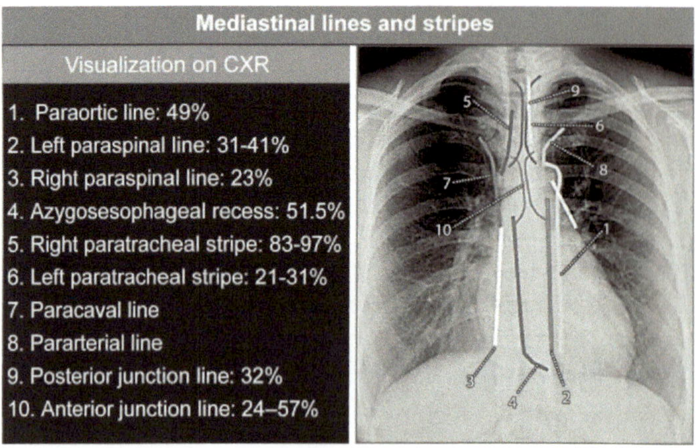

Fig. 2.37: Mediastinal lines.

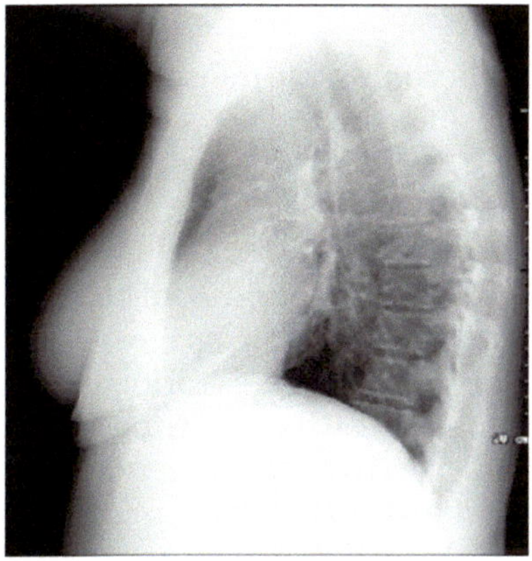

Fig. 2.38: Lateral x-ray.

- Retroclavicular regions
- Posterior mediastinal and paravertebral regions.

Mediastinal lines are described in the Figure 2.37.

How to Read a Lateral Film

When reading a patient's chest films you should look at both the PA and the lateral films.

Lateral chest X-ray can be taken with either the right or left side of the patient against the film.

Mount the film in such way that the vertebral column is on the right of you and the front of the chest is on the left of you, as shown in **Figure 2.38.**

Identify the Diaphragms

Right diaphragm can be seen to stretch across the whole thorax and can be seen clearly through the heart. Left diaphragm seems to disappear when it reaches the posterior border of heart. Gastric air bubble is seen closer to the left diaphragm. Posterior costophrenic angles are acute. Small amount of pleural fluid can blunt the CP angle.

Vertebral Translucency

Vertebral bodies become more translucent (darker) caudally. Loss of this translucency may be a sign of posterior basal segment pathology. Check the size, shape and density of vertebrae.

Compare the appearance of lung fields in front of and above the heart to those behind. They should be of equal density.

Look carefully at the clear spaces: retrosternal and retrocardiac spaces. These are areas of increased translucency corresponding to the site where both the lungs meet. Loss of translucency indicates pathology.

Normal retrosternal space measures 3 cm at its widest point. Retrosternal space obliterated in anterior mediastinal masses. Retrosternal space is widened in emphysema.

Check the position of fissures—horizontal and oblique fissure. Displacement, thickening of fissures has to be noted. Look for interlobar effusions.

Check the density of hila.

Trachea is seen to pass down in posterior direction to T6-T7 level. Posterior tracheal wall measures less than 5 mm (which includes tracheal and esophageal wall).

Soft tissues and bones have to be studied. Sternum and scapulae are well seen.

SILHOUETTE SIGN (FIGS. 2.39A AND B, TABLE 2.5)

One of the most useful signs in chest radiology is the silhouette sign. This was described by Dr Ben Felson. The silhouette sign is actually elimination of the silhouette or loss of lung/soft tissue interface caused by a mass or fluid in the normally air filled lung. For example, if an intrathoracic opacity is in anatomic contact with the heart border, then the opacity will obscure that border. The sign is commonly applied to the heart, aorta, chest wall, and diaphragm. The location of this abnormality can help to determine the location anatomically.

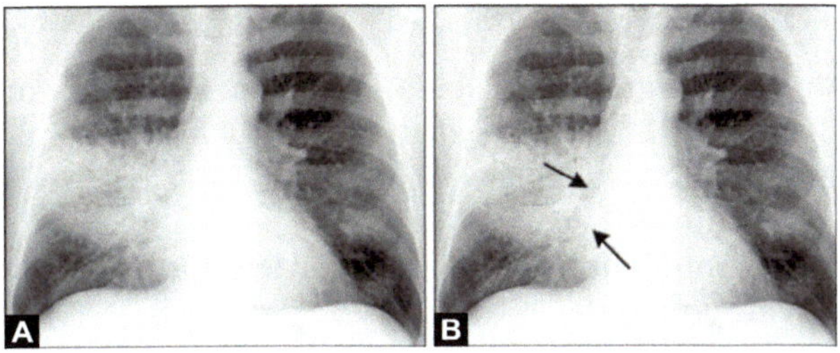

Figs. 2.39A and B: The right heart border is silhouetted out. This is caused by a pneumonia, involving the right middle lobe.

TABLE 2.5: Silhouetting structures and their contact with lungs.

Silhouette/structure	*Contact with lung*
» Upper right heart border/ ascending aorta	» Anterior segment of RUL
» Right heart border	» RML (medial)
» Upper left heart border	» Anterior segment of LUL
» Left heart border	» Lingula (anterior)
» Aortic knob	» Apical portion of LUL (posterior)
» Anterior hemidiaphragms	» Lower lobes (anterior)

Loss of right heart border

1. Right middle lobe atelectasis or airspace consolidation
2. Pleural disease
3. Mediastinal disease
4. Pectus excavatum
5. Scimitar syndrome

Loss of aortic knob

1. Left upper lobe disease
2. Mediastinal disease
3. Pleural disease

Loss of left heart border

1. Lingular collapse or airspace consolidation
2. Pleural disease
3. Mediastinal disease
4. Pericardial fat

Loss of hemidiaphragm

1. Lower lobe disease
2. Pleural disease

AIR BRONCHOGRAM (FIG. 2.40)

- Air bronchogram is a tubular outline of an airway made visible by filling of the surrounding alveoli by fluid or inflammatory exudates.
- It is diagnostic of consolidation.

Normal bronchi not usually visualized due to thin walls and an air-air interface.

Causes of air bronchograms are; consolidation, pulmonary edema, nonobstructive pulmonary atelectasis, severe interstitial disease, neoplasm and normal expiration.

CONSOLIDATION (FIG. 2.41)

Consolidation is defined as a process in which air in the alveoli is replaced by products of disease. The bronchi to the consolidated area are usually widely patent. In most instances, alveolar filling is patchy, i.e., not all acini are involved. The radiographic opacity is therefore nonhomogeneous, sometimes with air bronchogram. Causes include:

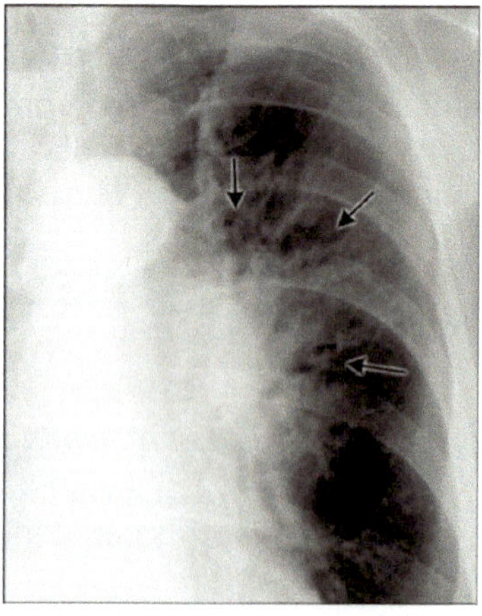

Fig. 2.40: Air bronchograms.

- **Pus:** Bacterial pneumonia
- **Blood:** Contusion, pulmonary hemorrhage
- **Water:** Pulmonary alveolar edema, aspiration
- **Cells:** Lymphoma, bronchioloalveolar cell carcinoma
- **Protein:** Pulmonary alveolar proteinosis

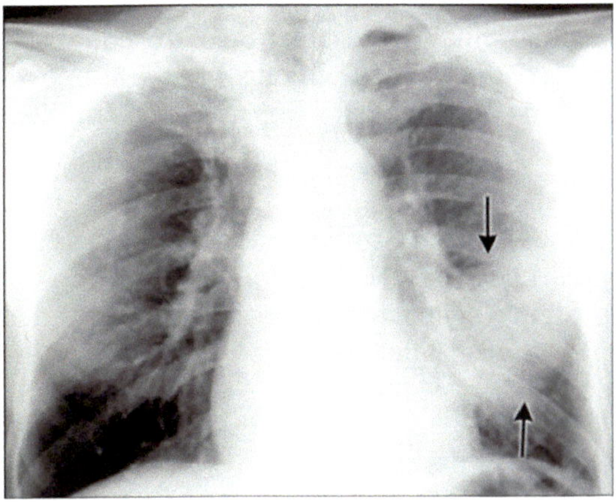

Fig. 2.41: Consolidation.

COLLAPSE (ATELECTASIS)

Atelectasis is volume loss due to alveolar collapse or failure to expand causing increased opacification of radiograph. Collapse may affect a whole lung or a subdivision (lobe, segment).

Types

- Obstructive
- Compressive
- Cicatrization
- Adhesive
- Passive.

General Features of Lobar Collapse

- Shift of fissures
- Area of increased opacity
- Crowding of vessels
- Tracheal displacement towards the side of the collapse
- Hilar shift
- Mediastinal shift towards the side of the collapse
- Elevation of the hemidiaphragm
- Herniation of the opposite lung across the midline.

Other Signs

- A hilar mass, which also suggests carcinoma as the cause.
- The presence of a foreign body
- The presence of an endotracheal tube; is it sited too low?
- Other evidence of malignant disease (e.g., rib metastases, effusion).

Collapse of Individual Lobes

Right Upper Lobe Collapse (Figs. 2.42 and 2.43)

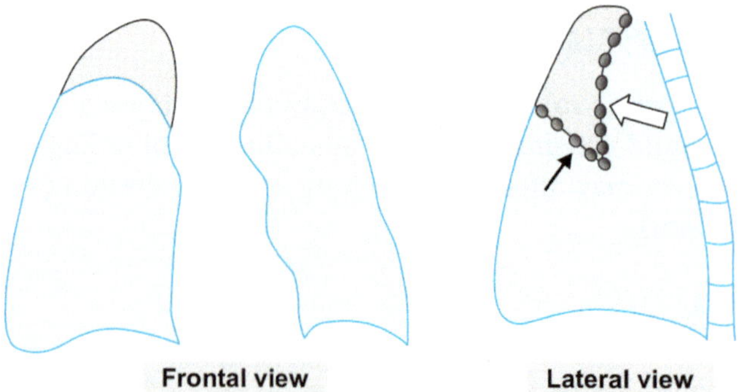

Fig. 2.42: The minor and major fissures move towards each other (black arrow = minor, white arrow = major).

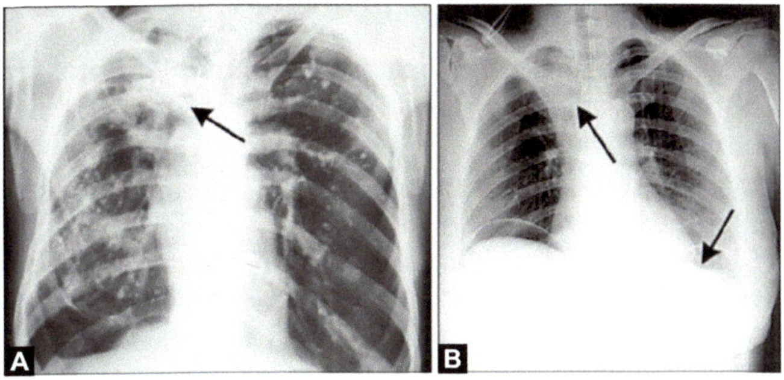

Figs. 2.43A and B: Examples of right upper lobe collapse; Incidental pneumoperitoneum seen in Figure B.

Signs of Right Upper Lobe Collapse

- Minor fissure moves upwards with concavity inferiorly.
- An area of opacity that lies against apex of mediastinum.
- Tracheal shift to the right.
- Right hilum is elevated and the intermediate bronchus assumes horizontal position.
- Loss of right paratracheal stripe (silhouette sign).

Right Middle Lobe Collapse (Fig. 2.44)

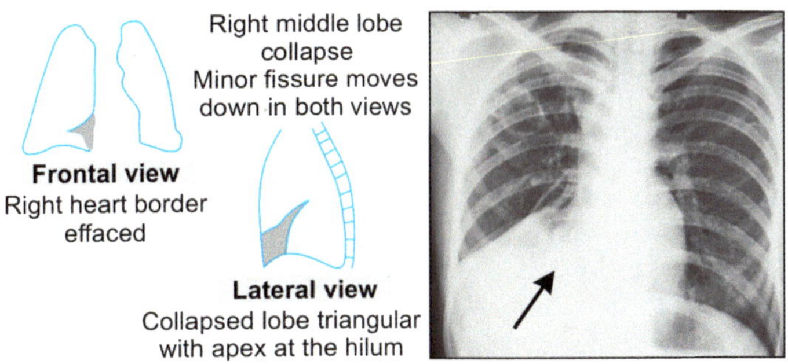

Fig. 2.44: Example of right middle lobe collapse.

Signs of Right Middle Lobe Collapse

- This is often not immediately obvious on the frontal film
- Ill-defined shadowing is evident adjacent to the right heart border, which becomes indistinct
- Right heart border is silhouetted
- Minor fissure moves downward
- Collapse of right middle lobe more obvious on lateral view
- In lateral view, collapsed lobe has triangular shape with apex at the hilum
- Also best seen in lordotic view.

Right Lower Lobe Collapse (Fig. 2.45)

Right lower zone shadowing is combined with obliteration of the hemidiaphragm (silhouette sign). The right heart border, which is anterior, is usually still clearly seen (silhouette sign again). The oblique fissure lies more horizontally and may become visible, giving a sharp upper margin to the shadowing. If the lobe collapses completely, it may appear as a triangular opacity behind the right heart border. The heart border, being anterior will still be clearly seen. On the lateral film there is abnormally increased density over the lower thoracic spine due to the triangular opacity of the collapsed lobe.

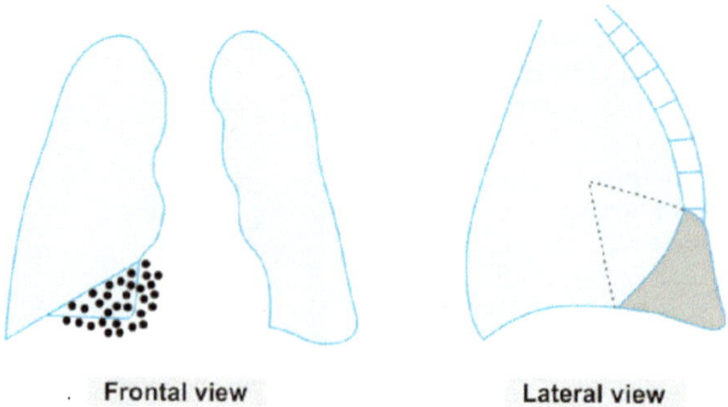

Fig. 2.45: Right lower lobe collapse. Opacity in the post-costophrenic angle. Major fissure moves backwards.

Left Upper Lobe Collapse (Figs. 2.46 and 2.47)

The left lung lacks a middle lobe and therefore a minor fissure, so left upper lobe atelectasis presents a different picture from that of the right upper lobe collapse. The result is predominantly anterior shift of the upper lobe in left upper lobe collapse, with loss of the left upper cardiac border. It casts a veil-like opacity over the left hemithorax, normally more dense towards the apex.

The expanded lower lobe will migrate to a location both superior and posterior to the upper lobe in order to occupy the vacated space and so the aortic knuckle characteristically remains clearly visible.

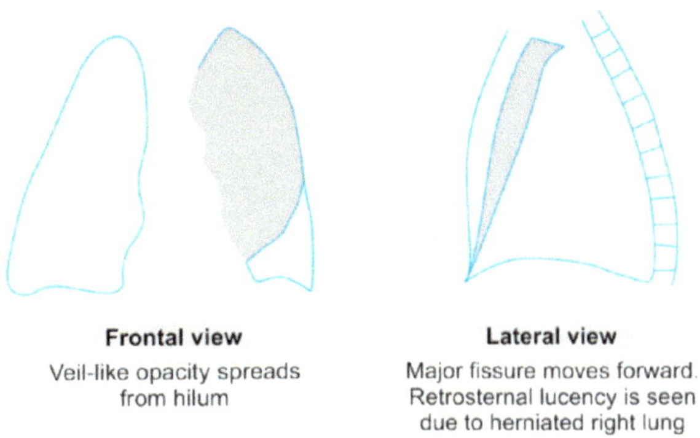

Fig. 2.46: Left upper lobe collapse.

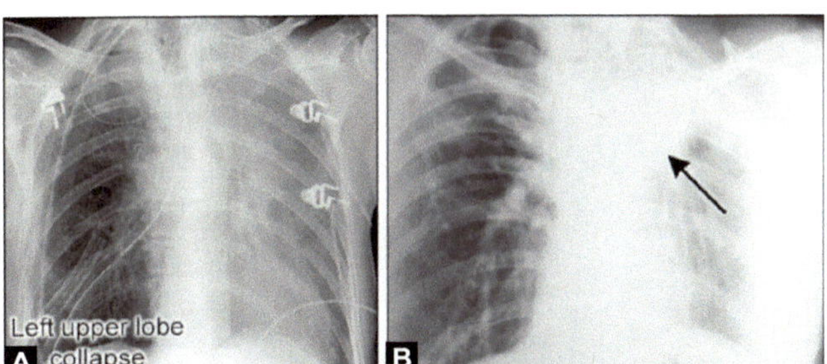

Figs. 2.47A and B: Examples of left upper lobe collapse.

Left Lower Lobe Collapse (Figs. 2.48 and 2.49)

The left lower lobe collapses medially and posteriorly to lie behind the heart. It classically displays a triangular opacity which may be visible through the cardiac shadow, or may overlie it, giving the heart an unusually straight lateral border. The hemidiaphragm may be obscured where the opacity lies against it. On the lateral film there is abnormally increased density over the lower thoracic spine due to the triangular opacity of the collapsed lobe.

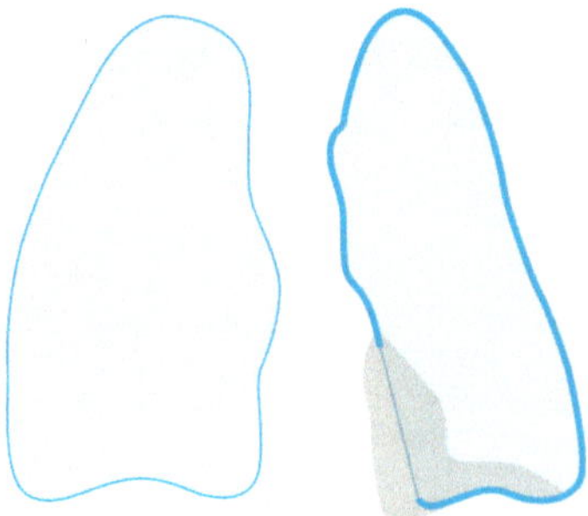

Frontal view

Fig. 2.48: Left lower lobe collapse.

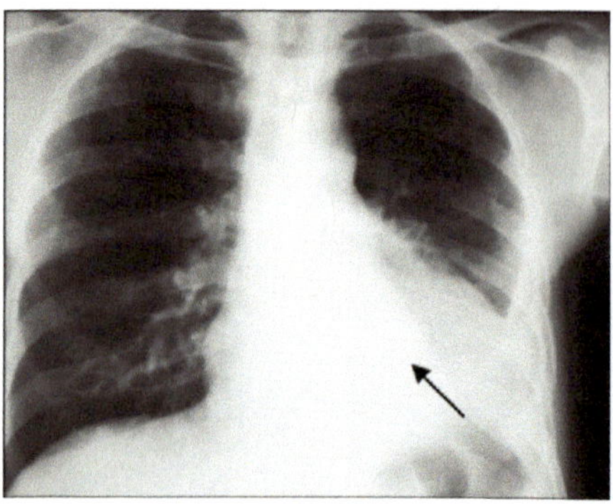

Fig. 2.49: Left lower lobe collapse.

Total Collapse of Lung (Figs. 2.50A and B)

Total collapse of a lung occurs when the obstruction is within the main stem bronchus. The appearance is one of total opacification of the affected hemithorax. The volume loss causes deviation of the trachea and shift of the mediastinum to the affected side. Sometimes the opposite lung may herniate across the midline, giving rise to the impression that some lung remains aerated. This is particularly so at the apices, at the site of the anterior and posterior junctional

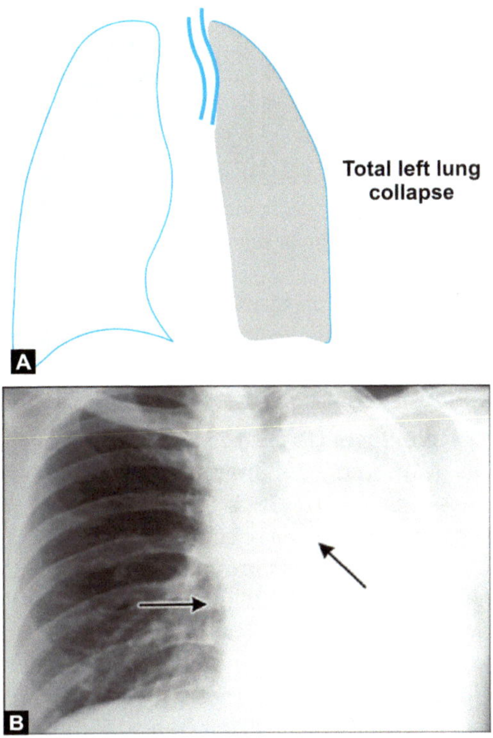

Figs. 2.50A and B: Total collapse of left lung.

lines. An effusion will produce midline shift in the opposite direction. However, collapse and effusion often coexist, in which case there may be minimal shift.

Segmental atelectasis (Figs. 2.51A and B): Appears as a wedge-shaped opacity with its apex at the hilum and its base in contact with the pleura. Other important features are fissural shift and positive silhouette sign. Sometimes it just appears as a narrow band of opacity.

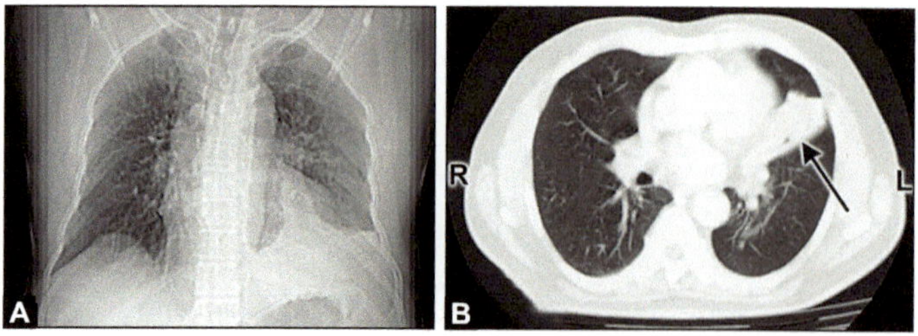

Figs. 2.51A and B: Digital scanogram and axial CT showing superior lingular segmental atelectasis.

Discoid atelectasis: Horizontal linear densities at the lung bases which usually make contact with the pleura. Associated with hypoventilation due to various causes. It's a common form of nonobstructive collapse.

Rounded atelectasis (RA): It is a form of nonsegmental peripheral pulmonary collapse that produces a pleural-based mass-like lesion. It is strongly associated with asbestos exposure. It is about 3-5 cm and is commonly located basally and dorsally and is composed of swirl of atelectatic parenchyma adjacent to thickened pleura. Other names are Blesovky's syndrome, helical atelectasis, pseudotumor, folded lung, etc. Conventional radiography may demonstrate rounded/oval subpleural opacity with vessels and airways converging towards the opacity in a helical fashion producing comet tail appearance **(Figs. 2.52A and B)**.

RA usually remains stable on serial radiologic studies, although very slow growth or regression may occur.

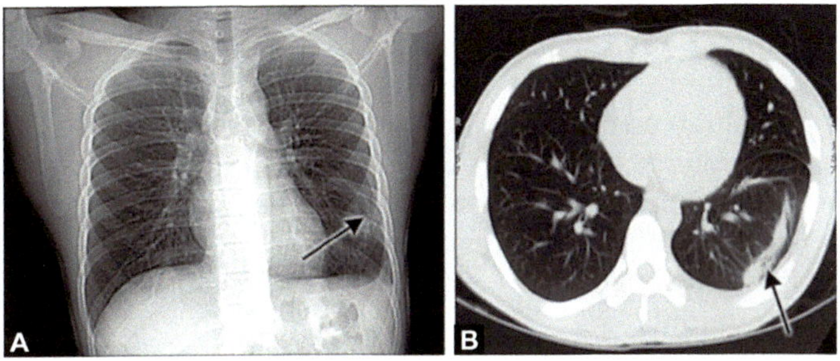

Figs. 2.52A and B: Digital scanogram and axial CT showing subpleural atelectasis with incurving of bronchovascular bundle.

X-ray imaging differences between atelectasis & pneumonia is summarised in **Table 2.6**.

TABLE 2.6: Major differentiating factors between atelectasis and pneumonia.

Atelectasis	*Pneumonia*
» Volume loss	» Normal or increased volume
» Associated ipsilateral shift	» No shift, or if present then contralateral
» Linear, wedge-shaped	» Consolidation, air space process
» Apex at hilum	» Not centered at hilum
Air bronchograms can occur in both	

PLEURAL DISEASE (FIGS. 2.53 TO 2.58)

Pleural Effusion

A pleural effusion is defined as fluid accumulating in the pleural space. The pleural space is a potential space lined by the visceral and parietal pleura. Normally less than

5 mL of free fluid is present in the pleural space. Excess pleural fluid accumulates when 1. Capillary hydrostatic pressure increases, 2. Blood oncotic pressure is low, 3. Capillary permeability is increased, and 4. Lymphatic obstruction.

The fluid can be transudative or exudative in nature. Terms used to refer to the various nature of effusions include:

- **Hydrothorax:** Transudative effusion, i.e., congestive heart failure (CHF), hypoalbuminemia
- **Pyothorax:** Pus in the pleural space, i.e., empyema from pneumonia
- **Hemothorax:** Blood
- **Chylothorax:** Chyle.

Malignant Effusion

Bilateral pleural effusions are usually transudates as they develop secondary to generalized systemic problems. Some of the bilateral effusions are exudates and are seen in metastatic disease, rheumatoid disease, lymphoma, SLE. Right-sided effusions are usually associated with ascites, heart failure, liver abscess. Left-sided effusions usually occur with pancreatitis, pericarditis, aortic dissection.

Radiological Signs of Pleural Effusion

The standard posterior-anterior (PA) and lateral chest radiographs remain the most important initial techniques for evaluating the pleural effusion. If fluid is free to distribute itself as influenced by gravity and elastic recoil of the lung, it will collect in the inferior hemithorax and between the inferior surface of the lung and the hemidiaphragm. Small effusions may fail to be detected because of the fluid's position in the posterior costophrenic gutters.

The standard PA radiograph can show changes with effusions as small as 250 mL. The lateral decubitus can sometimes distinguish very small effusions (15–25 mL). An effusion of 1 L will obscure the hemidiaphragm and extend up one-third to one-half of the hemithorax. As much as 200 to 300 mL may only cause blunting of the costophrenic angle laterally on the PA film.

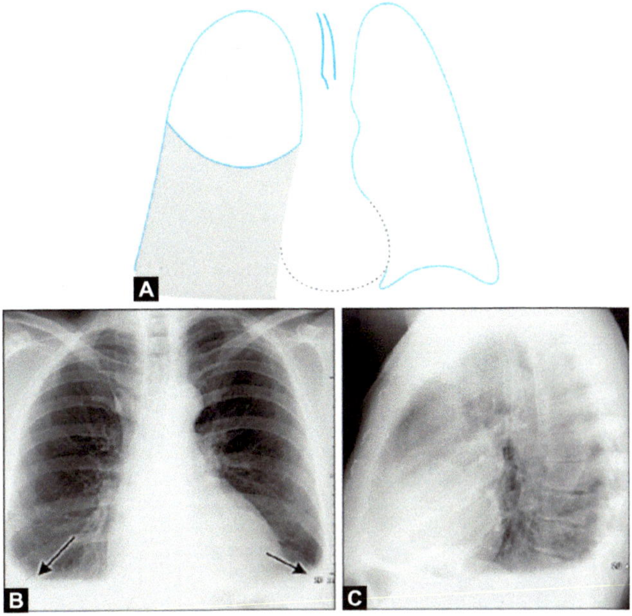

Figs. 2.53A to C: (A) Schematic showing right subpulmonic effusion; (B and C) CXR PA and lateral view showing bilateral pleural effusion. Note the blunting of CP angles with lateralization of the dome.

Larger effusions take on a typical pattern of (1) Homogeneous opacity over the lower hemithorax, (2) Obscuration of the hemidiaphragm, and (3) Concave upward border with the highest point along the lateral chest wall (meniscus).

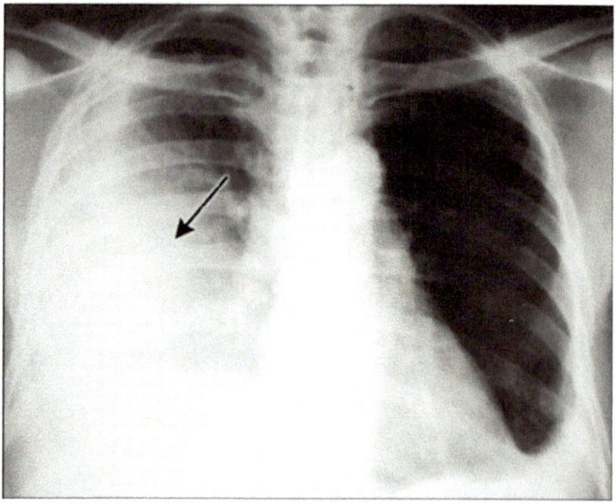

Fig. 2.54: CXR showing moderate right pleural effusion with mild left pleural effusion.

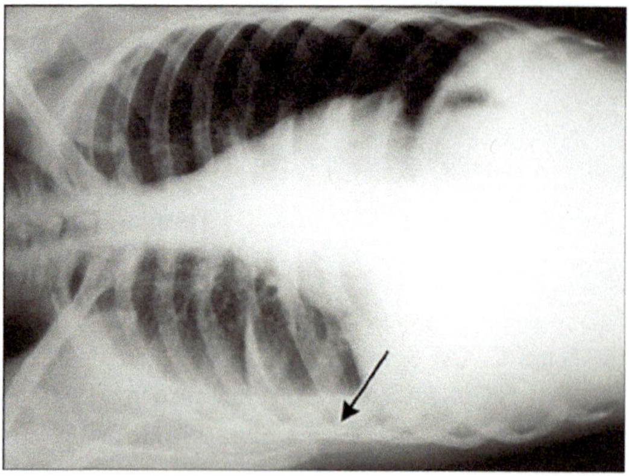

Fig. 2.55: The lateral decubitus X-ray uses the effect of gravity to help confirm the presence of free-flowing pleural fluid, especially small effusions.

Massive effusions cause opacification of hemithorax with shift of the mediastinum to the opposite side and sometimes inversion of ipsilateral diaphragm. Absence of mediastinal shift usually implies obstructive collapse of ipsilateral lung or pleural malignancy.

Causes of Opaque Hemithorax

- Pleural effusion
- Consolidation
- Collapse
- Massive tumor
- Fibrothorax
- Combination of above lesions
- Lung agenesis
- Pneumonectomy.

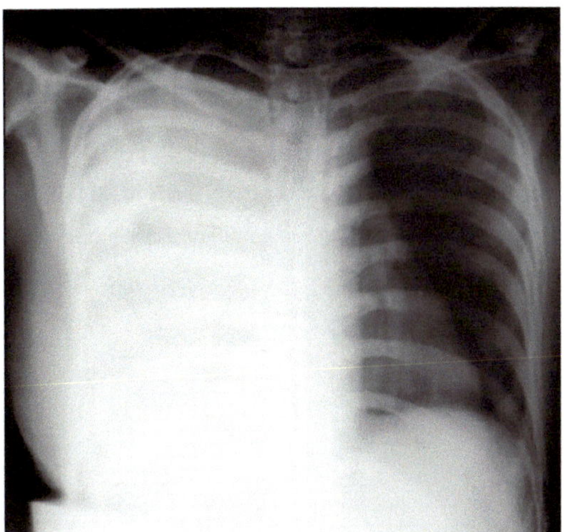

Fig. 2.56: Opaque right hemithorax.

Pleural Effusions in Supine Patient

Pleural effusions may also accumulate in the pleural space in an "atypical" distribution.

Subpulmonic Effusion (Fig. 2.53A)

Initially when there is minimal free pleural fluid, it will collect in the inferior hemithorax between the inferior surface of the lung and the hemidiaphragm. It will appear as an elevated hemidiaphragm with an unusual contour that peaks more laterally than usual and has a straight medial segment. A lateral decubitus X-ray is also valuable for confirming the presence of subpulmonic effusions. Left-sided subpulmonic effusions show increased separation between stomach gas and the hemidiaphragm.

Loculated Effusion (Figs. 2.57A and B)

Fluid at times becomes loculated in areas of the pleural space.

Fluid can loculate between visceral pleural layers in fissures or also between visceral and parietal layers of pleura.

Phantom tumor refers to fissural loculation of fluid, which commonly occurs in heart failure. These disappear with treatment and recur in the same place on repeated occasions.

Effusion can get loculated against chest wall, appearing as localized opacity convex to the lung with sharp edges.

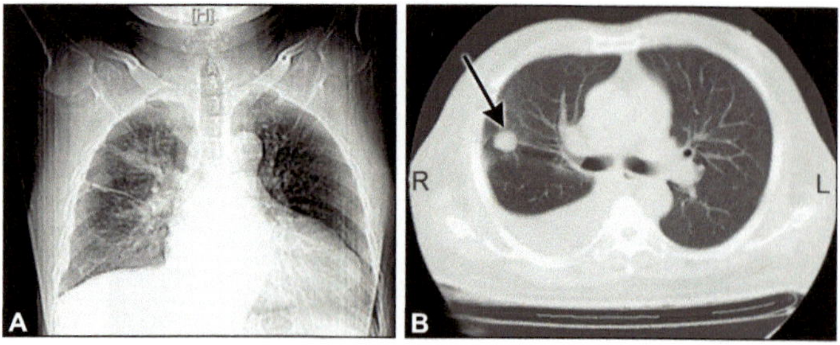

Figs. 2.57A and B: Loculated effusion in the right minor fissure (arrow).

Lamellar Effusion

In this the fluid gets collected between the lung and visceral pleura. It commonly occurs in cardiac failure. It is seen as a thin band of opacity between the lung and chest wall just above the costophrenic angle and is associated with septal lines.

Causes of Pleural Effusion

Transudate

- Congestive heart failure
- Renal failure
- Nephrotic syndrome
- Cirrhosis
- Superior vena cava syndrome
- Meigs syndrome.

Exudate

- Infection
- Neoplasia
- Pulmonary infarction
- Intra-abdominal process
- Collagen vascular diseases.

Hemorrhagic

- Neoplasia
- Tuberculosis
- Pulmonary infarction
- Trauma
- Iatrogenic.

Empyema

Pleural effusion with loculation.

The AP supine film is obtained when the patient is too ill for a standard PA and lateral exposure. It is much less than ideal.

PNEUMOTHORAX (FIGS. 2.59A AND B)

When air enters the pleural space, it is termed as pneumothorax. ***The two major categories are spontaneous***

pneumothoraces and traumatic (*See* **Table 2.7**) which develop after trauma. The spontaneous group is further divided into primary and secondary and the traumatic into iatrogenic and non-iatrogenic.

Primary spontaneous pneumothorax (PSP): The mechanism is felt to be the rupture of subpleural blebs in the lung, usually at the apices. The patients are usually male smokers who are tall and thin. Chest pain and dyspnea are the usual complaints and they are normally not a life-threatening occurrence. PSP occurs predominantly in young adults between 20–40 years.

Secondary spontaneous pneumothorax: There are many associated diseases, but chronic obstructive pulmonary disease and tuberculosis are the common causes.

Non-iatrogenic traumatic pneumothoraces are due to a variety of modes of injuries.

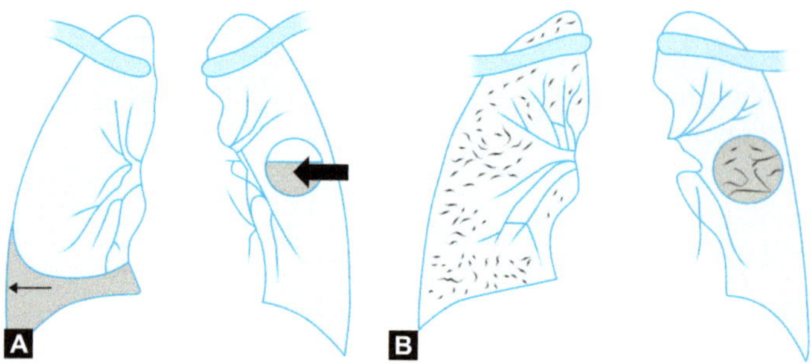

Figs. 2.58A and B: Comparison of upright and supine films. Schematics. (A) Upright PA chest film. Note the pleural effusion in the right hemithorax (black thin arrow) and (black thick arrow) the cavitary lesion with an air-fluid interface in the left lung; (B) Supine AP film, same subject. Note the changes in clavicular position, diaphragmatic height, mediastinal width, and distribution of blood flow. The pleural effusion now appears as a diffuse haziness on the right, and the cavitary lesion no longer shows the air-fluid interface.

Iatrogenic causes relate to invasive procedures and mechanical ventilation.

Catamenial pneumothorax is commonly a manifestation of endometriosis and is seen in women in their fourth decade. In these cases, pneumothoraces is recurrent occurring in relation to the menses and is predominantly right-sided and small.

Typical Signs

Typical signs of pneumothorax on an erect X-ray are:

Pneumothorax is seen as an area of transradiant zone without lung markings in the least dependent part of the chest. The visceral pleural line gets separated from the chest wall and is seen as white line of the pleura. In an upright film this is most likely seen in the apices. Lateral decubitus and expiratory film are helpful to diagnose small pneumothorax.

Partially collapsed lung may reveal clue to underlying cause of secondary pneumothorax and in primary pneumothorax the small apical blebs can be seen sometimes.

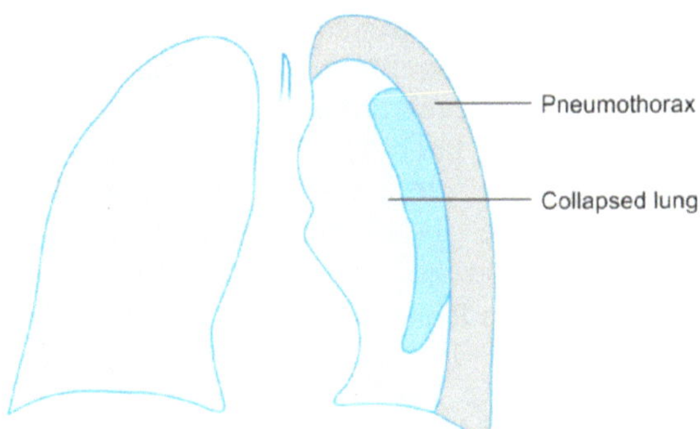

Fig. 2.59A: Schematic diagram depicting the effects of pneumothorax.

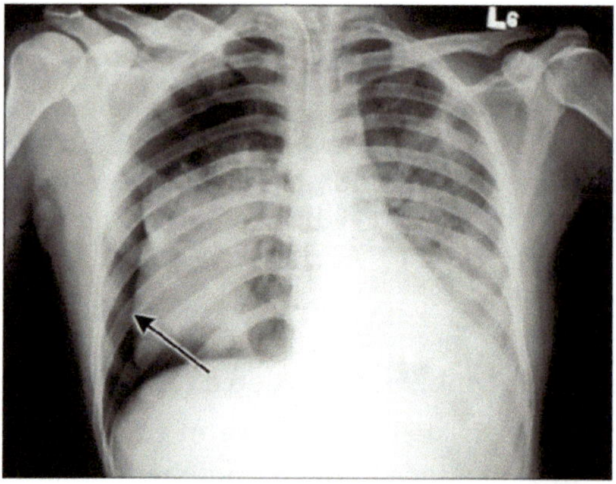

Fig. 2.59B: CXR PA view showing moderate right pneumothorax with collapse of right lung.

Atypical Signs

It can be difficult to see when the patient is in a supine position.

When the patient is in supine position air rises anteriorly and particularly to the medial aspect of the lung and may be seen as a lucency along the mediastinum. It may also collect in the inferior sulci causing a deep sulcus sign.

Signs that suggest pneumothorax in these conditions are: (1) Ipsilateral transradiancy, (2) Deep finger-like costophrenic sulcus laterally, (3) Anterior costophrenic recess seen as oblique line mimicking the adjacent diaphragm "double diaphragm sign", (4) Transradiant band against diaphragm and mediastinal border, and (5) Visualization of undersurface of heart and cardiac fat pads.

Hydropneumothorax (Figs. 2.60A and B)

A hydropneumothorax is both air and fluid in the pleural space. It is characterized by an air-fluid level on an upright or decubitus film in a patient with a pneumothorax. Some causes of a hydropneumothorax are trauma, thoracentesis, surgery, ruptured esophagus and empyema. **Figure 2.61** shows loculated hydropneumothorax.

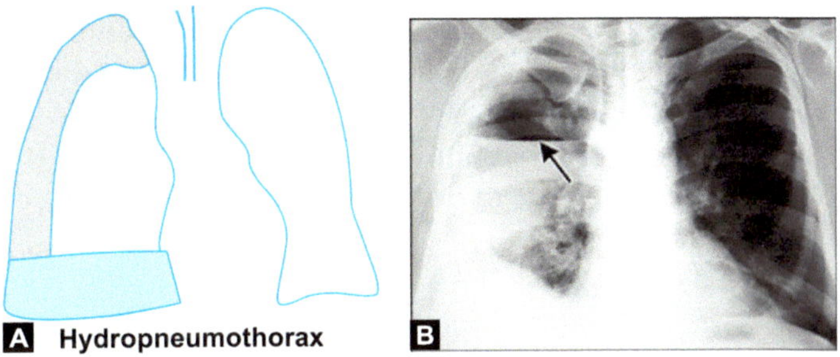

Figs. 2.60A and B: CXR showing right hydropneumothorax, note the air-fluid level.

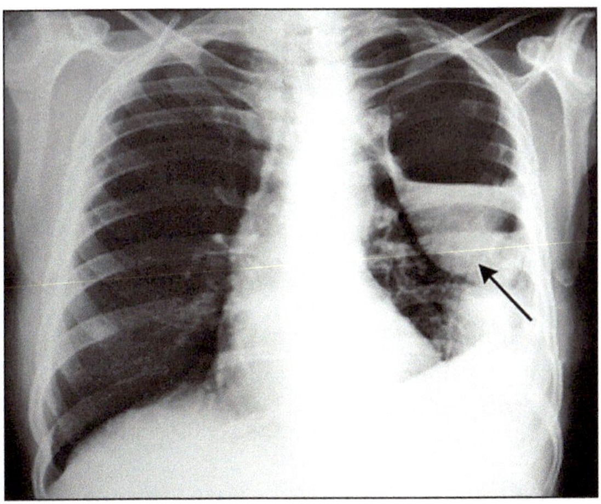

Fig. 2.61: CXR showing loculated left hydropneumothorax.

Tension Pneumothorax

It is a life-threatening complication. This leads to a build-up of air increasing intrathoracic pressure and eventually a positive pressure (tension pneumothorax) builds-up. The pressure build-up is large enough to collapse the lung and shift the mediastinum away from the pneumothorax. If it continues, it can compromise venous filling of the heart and even death.

A chest radiograph shows: (1) Transradiant hemithorax, (2) Mediastinal shift to opposite side **(Figs. 2.62A and B)**, (3) Ipsilateral diaphragm depression, and (4) Collapse of ipsilateral lung.

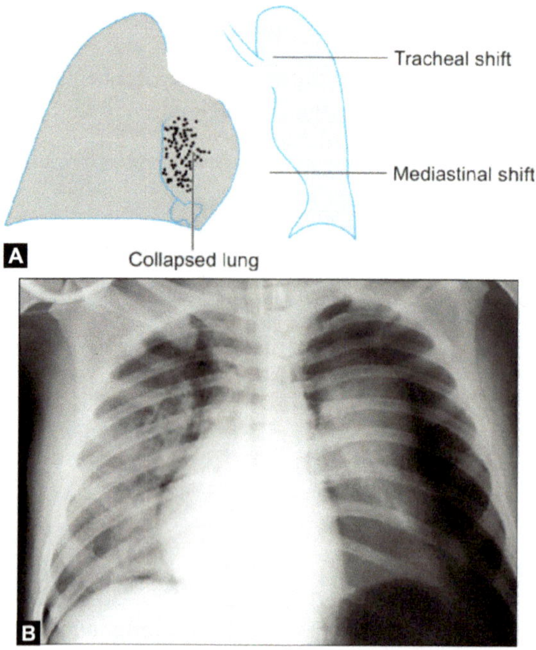

Figs. 2.62A and B: CXR showing bilateral pneumothorax with shift of mediastinum to the right.

Other Complications

Hemothorax: Associated with traumatic pneumothorax. Small amount of serous fluid or blood may accumulate. Blood may clot in pleural space and mimic a mass—fibrin body.

Pyopneumothorax is seen following necrotizing pneumonia or esophageal rupture.

TABLE 2.7: Causes of pneumothorax.

Spontaneous	
Primary	
Secondary	
Airflow obstruction	Asthma, COPD, cystic fibrosis
Pulmonary infection	Cavitary pneumonia, tuberculosis
	Fungal disease, AIDS
	Pneumatocele
Pulmonary infarction	
Neoplasm	Metastatic sarcoma
Diffuse lung disease	Histiocytosis X, lymphangioleio-myomatosis, fibrosing alveolitis, other diffuse fibroses
Heritable disorders	Marfan's syndrome
Endometriosis (catamenial pneumothorax)	
Traumatic	
Noniatrogenic	Ruptured esophagus/trachea, closed chest trauma (+/– rib fracture), Penetrating chest trauma
Iatrogenic	Thoracotomy/thoracocentesis, percutaneous biopsy, tracheostomy, central venous catheterization

Unilateral Hyperlucent Lung

- Chest wall deficiency
- Poland's syndrome
- Mastectomy
    - Obstructive emphysema
- MacLeod's syndrome
- Congenital absence of pulmonary artery
- Pulmonary thromboembolism
- Unilateral bullous emphysema
- Lobar collapse
- Pneumothorax
- Technical factors—rotated patient.

Pleural Calcification (Figs. 2.63A and B)

Pleural calcification is commonly seen in asbestos exposure, empyema, tuberculosis, hemothorax. In empyema the pleural calcifications are irregular and sheet-like with pleural thickening. It involves both parietal and visceral pleura. On en face images, they are seen as hazy veil-like dense opacities. In asbestos related pathology, the pleural calcifications are bilateral and discrete collections within the plaques. Usually involves parietal pleura.

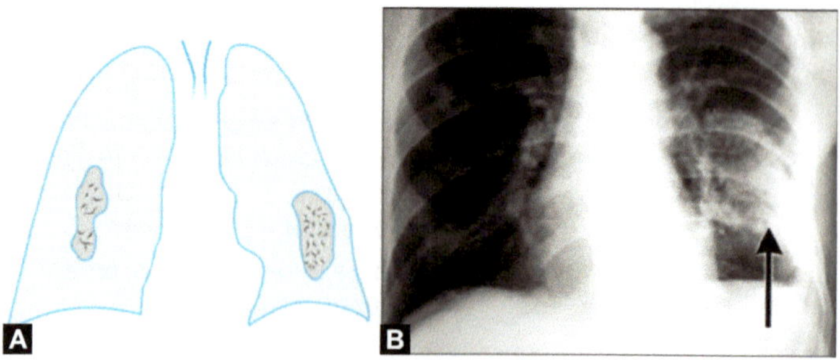

Figs. 2.63A and B: CXR showing confluent calcification of the left pleura.

Pleural Thickening (Fig. 2.64)

Pleural thickening can be localized or diffuse.

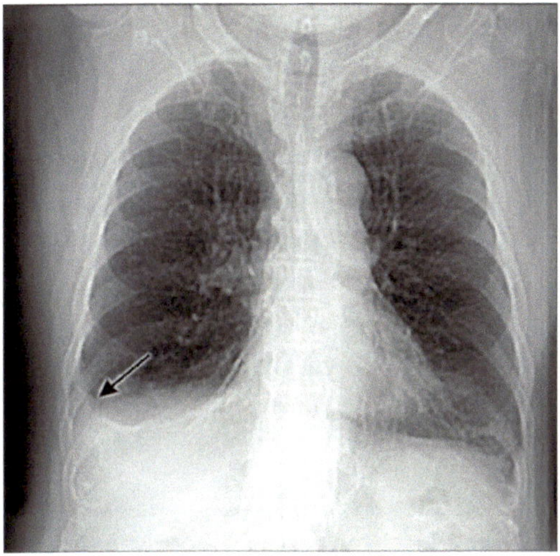

Fig. 2.64: CXR showing right basal pleural thickening.

Causes of Pleural Thickening

- Asbestos; talcosis
- Lung cancer (especially Pancoast tumor) mesothelioma **(Figs. 2.65A and B)**
- Metastatic disease
- Pleural effusion loculated
- Empyema (pyothorax)
- Old pleuritis, including TB
- Old trauma/surgery/hemothorax
- Fungus (histoplasmosis)
- Sarcoidosis
- Parasites.

Radiologically, pleural thickening produces soft tissue density shadowing, commonly seen in the dependent parts of the pleural cavity. Blunting of costophrenic angles is the common finding.

Apical pleural cap: These are pleural-based peripheral soft tissue opacities at the lung apex. They can be unilateral/bilateral. Usually seen in the elderly. Closest differential diagnosis is Pancoast tumor.

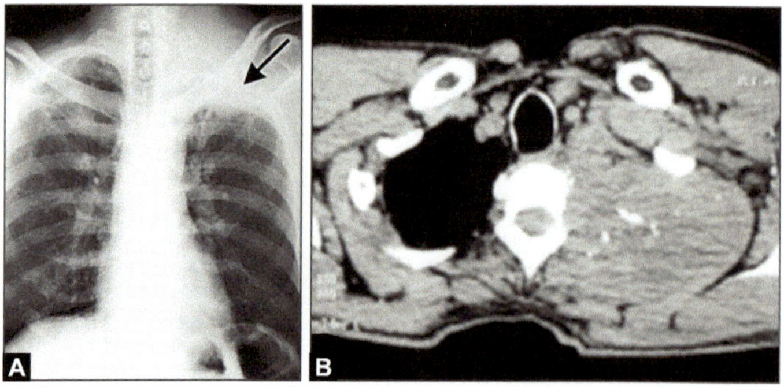

Figs. 2.65A and B: CXR and axial CT showing left upper apical opacity caused by Pancoast tumor.

Asbestos-related pleural plaque: These are well-defined soft tissue sheets originating from parietal pleura. They are usually bilateral and situated in the middle and lower zones and over the diaphragm. They usually calcify and give a "holly leaf" appearance with sharp angulated edges. Tangential views are helpful in diagnosing pleural plaques. Diffuse pleural thickening is less commonly seen than pleural plaques.

Pleural Thickening with Calcification

- Calcific fibrothorax, i.e., old hemothorax, old pyothorax/ tuberculous pleurisy
- Asbestos-related pleural disease
- Talc (pleurodesis)

- Rare:
  - Granulomatous infection (histoplasmosis)
  - Calcifying metastases (nodules, not thickening)
  - Calcifying parasitic disease.

Pleural Mass Lesions

Pleural-based Mass

- Lung cancer (likelihood depends on age and other risk factors)
- Focal infection/inflammation that is pleural-based
- Metastasis
- Benign spindle-cell tumor (lipoma, neurogenic tumor)
- Fibrous tumor of the pleura ("benign" mesothelioma)
- Loculated effusion/empyema
- Large (raised) pleural plaque
- Chest wall entities
- Remnants of old chest wall trauma
- **Chest wall tumor:** Askin tumor; sarcoma (osteosarcoma; chondrosarcoma).
- **Benign:** Aneurysmal bone cyst of rib.

Broad-based Pleural Opacity (Thickening) (Figs. 2.66A and B)

- Mesothelioma
- Metastasis
- Benign spindle-cell tumor (lipoma, neurogenic tumor)
- Loculated effusion/empyema
- Fibrothorax/chronic severe pleural thickening (post-inflammatory)
- Remnants of old chest wall trauma/old hematoma
- Postoperative changes, including flaps
- **Chest wall tumor:** Askin tumor; sarcoma (osteosarcoma; chondrosarcoma)

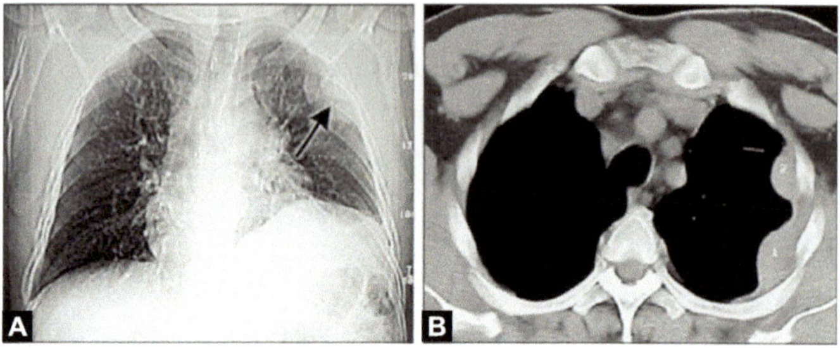

Figs. 2.66A and B: (A) CXR showing left upper zone pleural opacity; (B) Axial CT sections showing nodular pleural thickening.

- Large/thick pleural plaque
- Fibrous tumor of the pleura ("benign" mesothelioma)—more often mass-like than plaque-like.

Localized fibrous tumor (localized mesothelioma): These lesions are present in the middle age and are usually benign in nature. Few of them are malignant in nature (10%). These lesions have no relation with asbestos exposure. Radiologically they appear as solitary pleural based mass lesion which makes obtuse angle with the chest wall. It has lobulated margins and sometimes can be pedunculated. Associated hypertrophic osteoarthropathy can be present.

DIAPHRAGM

Eventration

It is caused due to absence of a part of muscle in the diaphragm which is replaced by a thin layer of connective tissue. It is usually associated with trisomies 13, 18, pulmonary hypoplasia, congenital cytomegalovirus (CMV). Eventration is more common on the left side.

Radiological features include:

- Hemidiaphragm not visualized
- Multicystic mass in the chest
- Mediastinal shift to opposite side.

Diaphragmatic Hernia

Morgagni Hernia (Figs. 2.67A and B)

Hernias through the foramen of Morgagni represent 2–3% of all diaphragmatic hernias. The defect is anterior and retrosternal in location and is usually a right-sided process. The contained contents may include, in order of decreasing frequency, the omentum, colon, stomach, liver, and small intestine. Morgagni hernia can be associated with trauma, severe effort, and obesity. On routine chest radiography, it usually appears as a rounded mass in the right cardiophrenic angle, adjacent to the anterior portion of the chest wall. The differential diagnosis includes pericardial fat pad, pericardial cyst, or solid tumor.

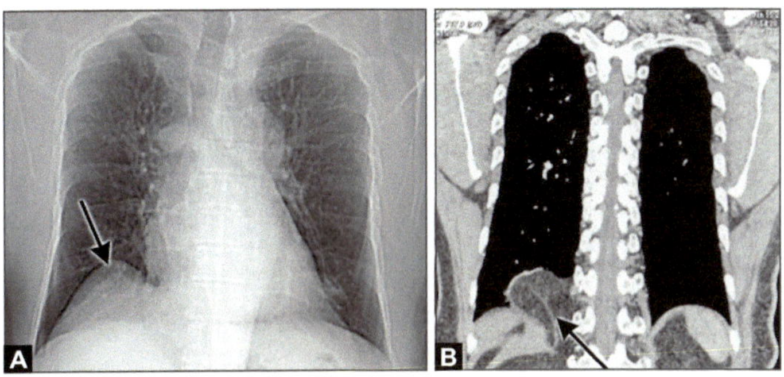

Figs. 2.67A and B: Digital scanogram showing right diaphragmatic hump-like opacity, coronal reconstructions showing herniation of fat through the diaphragmatic defect.

Bochdalek Hernia (Fig. 2.68)

Hernias through the foramen of Bochdalek are developmental defects in the posterior part of the diaphragm. These hernias are usually diagnosed in infants who present with clinical symptoms of pulmonary insufficiency. The herniated contents contain fat and omental tissue in a majority of cases, and also retroperitoneal and intraperitoneal structures can be involved. Left-sided hernias are more common. On conventional radiographs, the hernia may appear as a lung-base soft-tissue-opacity lesion seen posteriorly on lateral images.

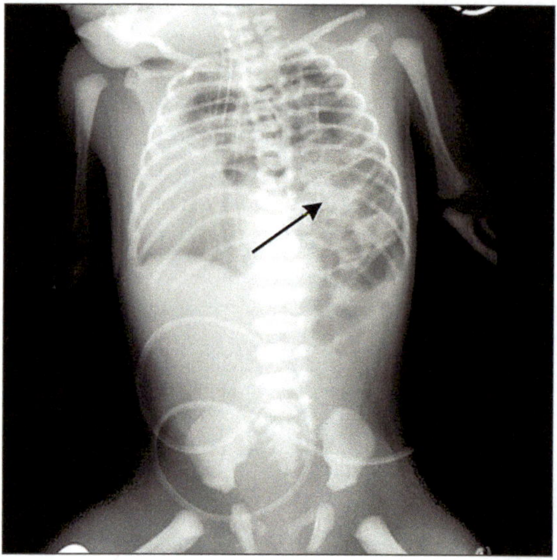

Fig. 2.68: CXR showing scaphoid abdomen with bowel loops in the left chest causing mediastinal shift.

Hiatal Hernia

Hiatal hernias may be ***sliding or paraesophageal*** (less common). Sliding hernias involve upward displacement of the esophageal junction through the esophageal hiatus in the diaphragm into the posterior mediastinum. Paraesophageal hernias involve protrusion of the stomach into the thorax through the esophageal hiatus. On chest radiographs, a paraesophageal hernia may appear as a soft-tissue-opacity lesion posterior to the heart near the esophageal hiatus.

Diaphragmatic Injury (Figs. 2.69A and B)

Diaphragmatic injuries occur in 0.8–8% of patients after blunt trauma. Diaphragmatic injuries remain a diagnostic challenge for both radiologists and surgeons. In most cases, the diagnosis may be obvious at chest radiography and computed tomography (CT); however, some specific signs require careful analysis with CT and magnetic resonance (MR) imaging.

Injuries to the left hemidiaphragm occur three times more frequently than injuries to the right side following blunt trauma, possibly due to a buffering effect of the liver on the right hemidiaphragm. Both bilateral tears and extension of tears into the central tendon are uncommon. Mechanisms of injuries include a lateral impact, which distorts the chest wall and shears the diaphragm, and a direct frontal impact, which leads to increased intra-abdominal pressure. Most ruptures are longer than 10 cm and occur at the posterolateral aspect of the hemidiaphragm between the lumbar and intercostal attachments. This is the weakest point of the diaphragm, where the pleuroperitoneal membrane finally closes at embryogenesis. Ruptures of the diaphragm can also occur in its central portion and at its costal attachment.

Penetrating injuries produce small diaphragmatic holes, which are often overlooked.

Common associated injuries include pelvic fractures, splenic injuries, and renal injuries. There is also a high frequency of liver injuries. Thoracic injuries such as pneumothoraces/hemothoraces and rib fractures are seen commonly.

Chest radiography remains valuable in the acute phase for the detection of diaphragmatic rupture. Right diaphragmatic injuries are more difficult to detect on radiographs. The liver serves to block herniation of

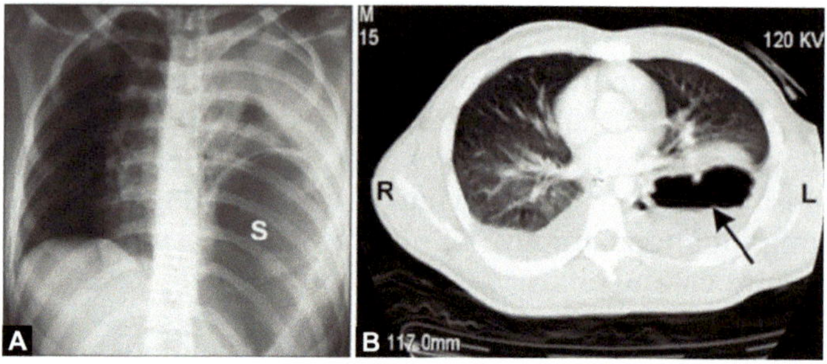

Figs. 2.69A and B: (A) CXR showing dilated stomach herniating into left hemithorax following a road traffic accident; (B) Axial CT showing the intrathoracic stomach.

abdominal contents into the lower right side of the chest. Herniation of the liver is often overlooked. Findings of diaphragmatic tears on chest radiographs include the following: (1) Intrathoracic herniation of a hollow viscus (stomach, colon, small bowel) with or without focal constriction of the viscus at the site of the tear—***collar sign*** and (2) Visualization of a nasogastric tube above the hemidiaphragm on the left side.

Findings suggestive of hemidiaphragmatic rupture include elevation of the hemidiaphragm, distortion or obliteration of the outline of the hemidiaphragm, and contralateral shift of the mediastinum.

Other associated findings related to the trauma such as pleural effusion, pulmonary contusion or laceration, atelectasis, and phrenic nerve palsy can mimic or mask diaphragmatic injury on chest radiographs.

Unilateral Elevated Hemidiaphragm

- Causes above the diaphragm:
  - Pulmonary collapse
  - Phrenic nerve palsy

  - Pulmonary hypoplasia
  - Pulmonary thromboembolism
  - Pleurisy.
- Diaphragmatic causes:
  - Eventration
  - Trauma.
- Causes below the diaphragm:
  - Gaseous distension of stomach
  - Subphrenic mass/abscess
  - Hepatic/splenic abscess.
- Scoliosis
- Posture—lateral decubitus (dependent side)

Bilateral Elevated Diaphragms

- Causes above the diaphragms
  - Bilateral pulmonary collapse
  - Diffuse pulmonary fibrosis
- Causes below the diaphragm
  - Ascites
  - Pregnancy
  - Pneumoperitoneum
  - Hepatosplenomegaly
  - Large intra-abdominal tumor
  - Intestinal obstruction
  - Post abdominal surgery
- Diaphragmatic causes
  - Bilateral diaphragmatic paralysis
- Poor inspiratory effort
- Obesity.

PNEUMOMEDIASTINUM (FIGS. 2.70 AND 2.71)

Pneumomediastinum may result from a variety of causes that may be either intrathoracic (e.g., narrowed or plugged airway, straining against a closed glottis, blunt chest trauma, alveolar

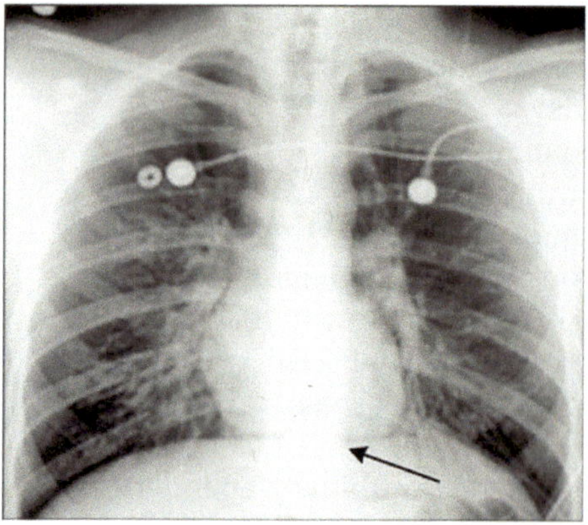

Fig. 2.70: CXR showing continuous diaphragm sign of pneumomediastinum.

rupture) or extrathoracic (e.g., sinus fracture, iatrogenic manipulation in dental extraction, perforation of a hollow viscus). The radiographic signs of pneumomediastinum depend on the depiction of normal anatomic structures that are outlined by the air as it leaves the mediastinum. These signs include the thymic sail sign, "ring around the artery" sign, tubular artery sign, double bronchial wall sign, **continuous diaphragm sign (Fig. 2.70)**, and extrapleural sign. In distal esophageal rupture, air may migrate from the mediastinum into the pulmonary ligament. Pneumomediastinum may be difficult to differentiate from medial pneumothorax and pneumopericardium. Occasionally, normal anatomic structures (e.g., major fissure, anterior junction line) may simulate air within the mediastinum.

BASICS OF CARDIAC DIAGNOSIS FROM CHEST X-RAY (FIGS. 2.72 TO 2.77)

The first observation usually made is that of the heart size: The cardiothoracic ratio.

Heart Size (Fig. 2.72)

The cardiothoracic ratio is the maximum transverse diameter of the heart divided by the greatest internal diameter of the thoracic cage (from inside of rib to inside of rib).

In normal people, the cardiothoracic ratio is usually less than 50%. Therefore, the cardiothoracic ratio is a handy way of separating most normal hearts from most abnormal hearts.

But it is not without pitfalls. A heart may be greater than 50% of the cardiothoracic ratio and still be a normal heart.

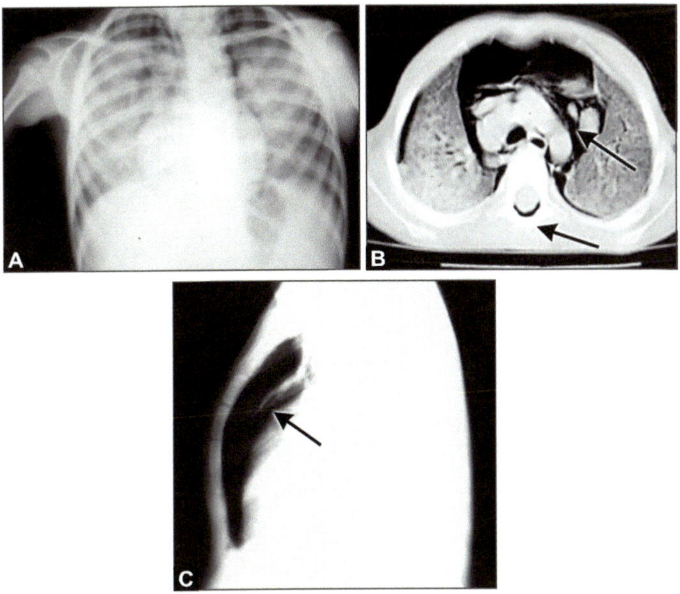

Figs. 2.71A to C: (A) CXR showing bilateral pneumothorax and pneumomediastinum; (B) Axial CT section showing pneumomediastinum and pneumorachis. Lungs appear white due to acute interstitial pneumonia; (C) Lateral X-ray showing increased anterior mediastinal lucency.

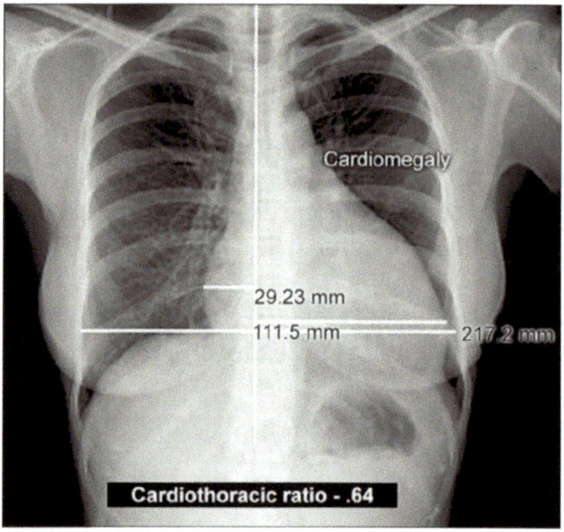

Fig. 2.72: Method of measuring CTR.

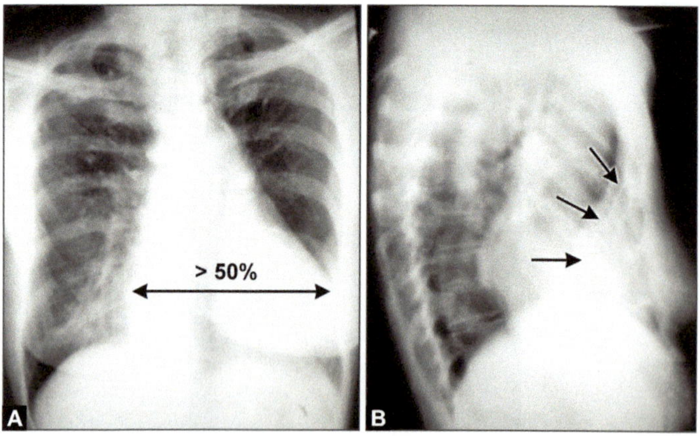

Figs. 2.73A and B: Pectus excavatum deformity causing pseudocardiomegaly.

This can occur if there is an extracardiac cause of cardiac enlargement. Extracardiac causes of cardiac enlargement include:

Inability to take a deep breath because of:
- Obesity
- Pregnancy, or
- Ascites

Or abnormalities of the chest that compress the heart such as:
- Pectus excavatum deformity **(Figs. 2.73A and B)**, or
- Straight back syndrome

Sometimes the heart can be smaller than 50% of the cardiothoracic ratio but still be an abnormal heart. This occurs when there is something obstructing the flow of blood from the ventricles since the ventricles respond at first by undergoing hypertrophy, which does not produce cardiomegaly.

Since not all abnormal hearts are enlarged, definition of cardiac disease in those individuals depends on an assessment of the contours of the heart on the frontal film.

Cardiac Contours (Fig. 2.74)

1. On the right side of the heart, the first contour is that of the ascending aorta.
   This is a low density, almost-straight edge visible just to the right of the trachea anatomically representing the superior vena cava and the brachiocephalic vein but in practice reflecting the size of the ascending aorta. So we shall call this contour the ascending aorta.
   The ascending aorta can be small as in ASD or it can be convex outward as in aortic stenosis, aortic regurgitation, and hypertensive cardiovascular disease. The ascending aorta should never project farther to the right than the right heart border in a normal person.
2. Just below the ascending aorta is an indentation where the so-called "double density of left atrial enlargement" will appear when the left atrium enlarges toward the right side of the heart.

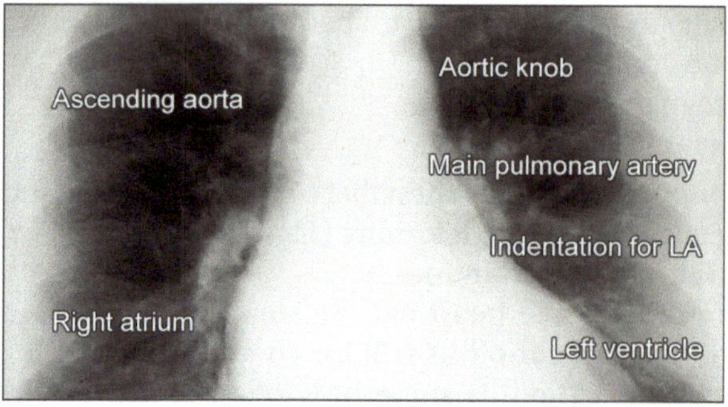

Fig. 2.74: Normal cardiac contours.

Normally, the left atrium forms no border of the heart in the frontal projection. When the left atrium enlarges, it may produce two abnormal contours of the heart.

Where the ascending aorta meets the right atrium, there is usually an indentation. In patients with an enlarged left atrium which projects to the right, there will be two overlapping densities seen where this indentation normally is. One of the densities is the normal right atrium. The other overlapping density is the enlarged left atrium. The double density may occasionally be seen in normal individuals; always check left heart border for straightening **(Fig. 2.80)**.

3. The last contour on the right side of the heart is the right atrium. In an adult, every disease that causes enlargement of the right atrium also produces enlargement of the right ventricle **(Fig. 2.75)**. So we can consider the right atrium and ventricle together as a single functional unit in adults and we will estimate right-sided cardiac enlargement by observing another cardiac contour, but not the right atrium. Therefore, for this system the right atrium is not an important contour.

   Now we move to the left heart border and start at the top.

4. On the left side of the heart, the first contour is the aortic knob. The aortic knob is a radiographic structure that is formed by the foreshortened aortic arch and a portion of the descending aorta.
   In normal people the aortic knob measures less than 35 mm when measured from the lateral border of the trachea to the lateral border of the aortic knob.
   The knob will be greater than 35 mm due to increased pressure, flow, or changes in the elasticity of the wall, e.g., cystic medial necrosis, dissection of the aorta.
5. Just below the aortic knob is the main or undivided segment of the pulmonary artery. The main pulmonary is very important in this system and forms the cornerstone for two of the main categories of disease to follow.
   First, you must be able to find the main pulmonary artery segment. Then, you can measure it.
   You can find the main pulmonary artery by either locating the first contour below the aortic knob or by finding the adjacent squiggly vessels that are the left pulmonary artery. The main and left pulmonary arteries are always adjacent to each other.
   We can measure the main pulmonary artery by drawing a tangent line from the apex of the left ventricle to the aortic knob and then measuring along a perpendicular to that tangent line, the distance between the tangent and the main pulmonary artery.
   In normal people, the distance between the tangent and the main pulmonary artery lies within a range of values between 0 mm (the main pulmonary is touching the tangent line) to as far away from the tangent line (medially) as 15 mm **(Fig. 2.76)**. Therefore, this sets up two major categories of abnormality. First, the main pulmonary artery may project beyond the tangent line (greater than 0 mm). This can occur if there is increased pressure or increased flow in the pulmonary circuit.

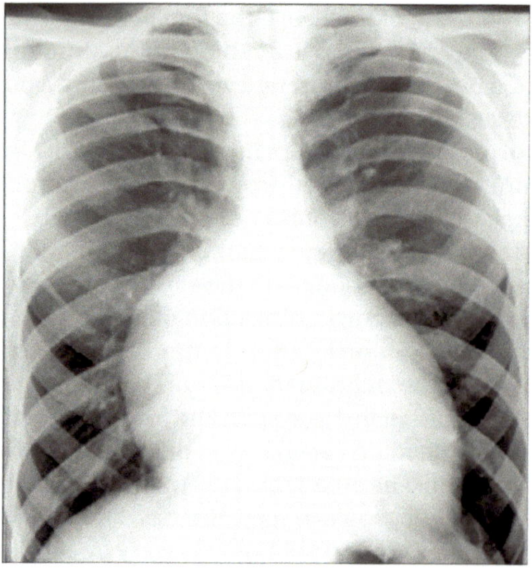

Fig. 2.75: Enlarged RA seen in Ebstein's anomaly.

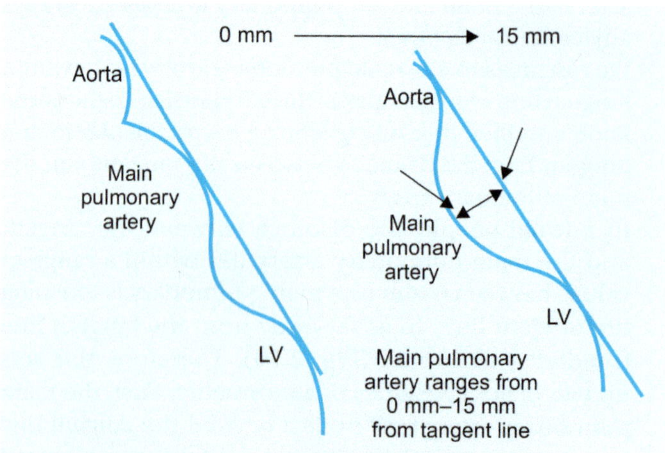

Fig. 2.76: Scheme showing the MPA measurement.

Second, the main pulmonary artery may project more than 15 mm away from the tangent line. This can occur either because there is something intrinsically wrong with the pulmonary artery such as absence or hypoplasia of the pulmonary artery, e.g., Tetralogy of Fallot, truncus. But, these diseases are uncommon in adults.

The other reason the main pulmonary artery may be more than 15 mm from the tangent line is the left ventricle and/ or aortic knob may enlarge and push the tangent line away from pulmonary artery, e.g., atherosclerosis. These are very common diseases.

Young females may normally have prominence of the MPA but rarely does the main pulmonary artery project beyond the tangent.

6. Just below the main pulmonary artery segment (area between the main pulmonary artery and the left ventricle) is a little concavity where the left atrium, when it enlarges on the left side of the heart, will appear.

   Filling in at this concavity by an enlarged left atrium produces "straightening" of the left heart border **(*see* Fig. 2.83)**. It may be seen in mitral disease or shunt (VSD, PDA) and rarely left atrial myxoma, papillary muscle dysfunction and chronic heart failure.

   Sometimes, the left atrial appendage may enlarge as well. A convexity at this contour means the left atrial appendage is enlarged and is seen in mitral valvular disease, usually mitral stenosis.

7. The last cardiac contour is the **left ventricle**.

   The best way to evaluate which ventricle is enlarged (i.e. right or left) is to look at the corresponding outflow tracts for each ventricle.

   If the heart is enlarged and the main pulmonary artery is large (sticks out beyond the tangent line), then the cardiomegaly is made up of at least right ventricular enlargement.

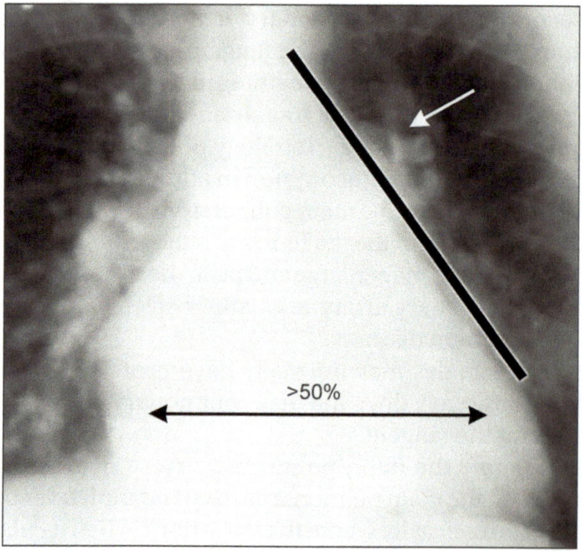

Fig. 2.77: X-ray showing cardiomegaly with enlarged MPA suggesting RV enlargement as a cause for cardiomegaly.

If the heart is enlarged and the aorta is prominent (ascending, knob, descending), then the cardiomegaly is made up of at least left ventricular enlargement **(Fig. 2.77)**.

Once one ventricle is determined to be enlarged, then the other ventricle may also be enlarged but there is no way to identify this with a chest X-ray.

Pulmonary Vasculature (Figs. 2.78 and 2.79)

It is important to know that the pulmonary vasculature will fall into one of the following four categories:

1. Normal
2. Pulmonary venous hypertension
3. Pulmonary arterial hypertension
4. Increased flow.

1. **Measure the right descending pulmonary artery (RDPA):** The RDPA is visible on almost all chest films as a large vessel just to the right of the right heart border. Its diameter can be measured at about the level of the indentation between the ascending aorta and the right atrium.
   In normal people, **the right descending pulmonary artery is less the 17 mm in diameter**.
2. **Evaluate the distribution of flow from apex to base:** In normal people, in the erect position, the blood flow to the bases is greater than the blood flow to the apices. This is due to the effect of gravity. In normal people, the size of the vessels at the base will therefore be greater than the size of the vessels at the apex.
   In people with **pulmonary venous hypertension**, the blood flow to the apex becomes equal to or greater than the blood flow to the base. Therefore, the size of the vessels at the apex becomes equal to or greater than the size of the vessels at the bases—a reversal of the normal distribution pattern. This is known as **cephalization**.
3. **Evaluate the distribution of flow from central to peripheral:** Normally, the pulmonary vessels taper gradually from central to peripheral. It does not matter whether they are arteries or veins and it does not matter whether it is the lung or any other organ, blood vessels taper gradually from central to peripheral.

In **pulmonary arterial hypertension**, there is a re-distribution of flow in the lungs from central to peripheral such that the peripheral vessels appear too small for the size of the central vessels from which they come. This discrepancy in the size of the central pulmonary vessels (which are large) compared to the peripheral pulmonary vasculature (which even though it is small is still indistinguishable from normal) is called **pruning**.

Using the size of the RDPA and the distribution of flow in the lungs—apex to base and central to peripheral, we can define the four states of the pulmonary vasculature.

Normal Pulmonary Vasculature

- The right descending pulmonary artery is less than 17 mm.
- The lower lobe vessels are larger than the upper lobe vessels.
- There is a gradual tapering of the blood vessels from central to peripheral.

Pulmonary Venous Hypertension

- The right descending pulmonary artery is usually greater than 17 mm.
- The upper lobe vessels are equal to or greater than the size of the lower lobe vessels (cephalization).
- There is a gradual tapering of the blood vessels from central to peripheral.

Pulmonary Arterial Hypertension

- The right descending pulmonary artery is greater than 17 mm.
- The lower lobe vessels are larger than the upper lobe vessels.
- There is a rapid decrease in the size of the peripheral vessels relative to the central vessels from which they come (pruning).

Increased Flow

- The right descending pulmonary artery is greater than 17 mm.
- The lower lobe vessels are larger than the upper lobe vessels.
- There is a gradual tapering of the blood vessels from central to peripheral.

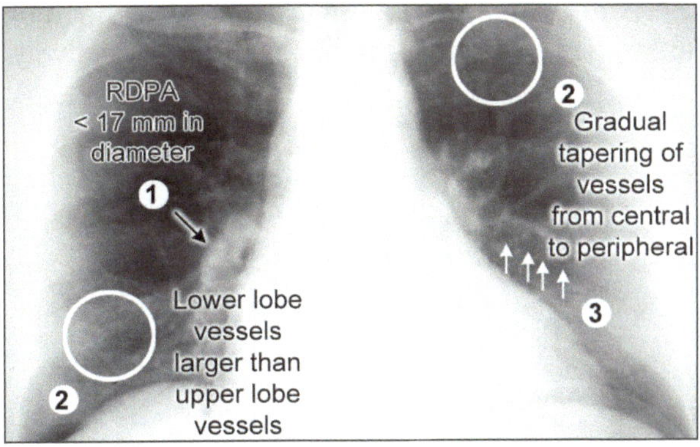

Fig. 2.78: Schematic diagram showing the normal pattern of pulmonary vessels.

A. Normal pulmonary flow
- Gradual and smooth branching pattern
- Caudalization at rest
- Right descending pulmonary artery 10–15 mm for males. 9–14 mm for females. Values > 1 mm outside the limits are abnormal
- Artery-bronchus ratio = 1.2:1, larger or smaller arteries are abnormal

↓

B. Cephalization of pulmonary vessels—post-capillary PHT
- Centralization—precapillary PHT
- Lateralization—unilateral increase in PHT

↓

C. Large pulmonary artery and vein—increase flow (ASD)
- Pulmonary artery larger than vein—hypertension
- Large artery, vein and wide pedicle—increased volume (renal failure)

Fig. 2.79: Flowchart showing a basic classroom approach.

Figures 2.80 and **2.81** show straightening of left heart border and enlargement of left pulmonary artery, respectively.

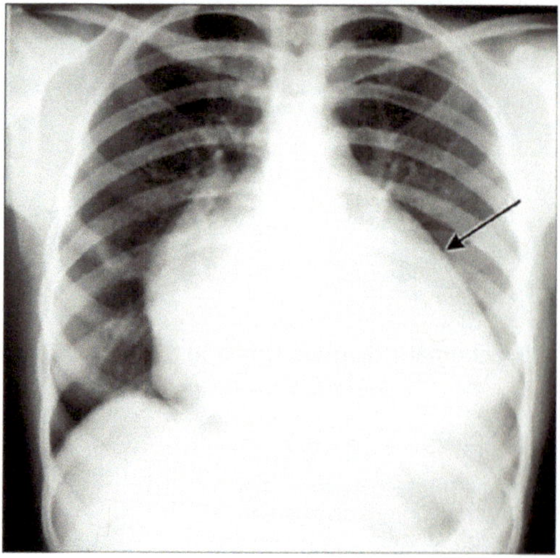

Fig. 2.80: CXR showing straightening of left cardiac border.

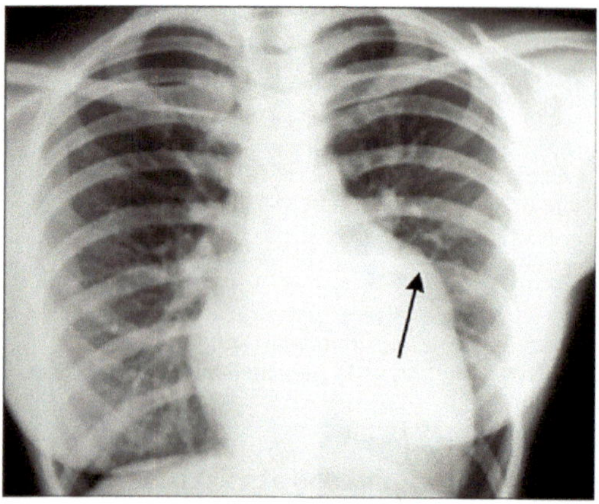

Fig. 2.81: CXR showing enlarged left pulmonary artery.

Figure 2.82 shows chest x-ray having enlarged right descending pulmonary artery and enlarged left pulmonary artery in a patient with pulmonary hypertension.

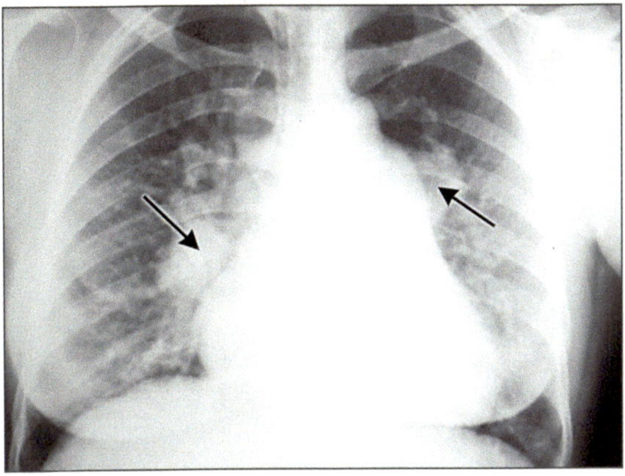

Fig. 2.82: CXR showing enlargement of RDPA and left pulmonary artery.

Figures 2.83A and B shows PA view & lateral view of chest x-ray having calcified of left ventricular aneurysm respectively.

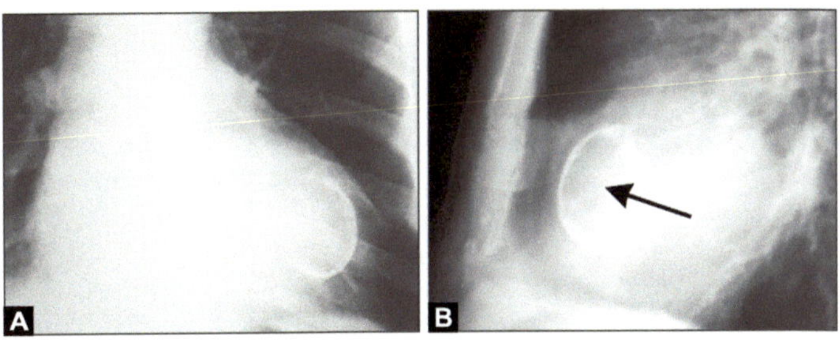

Figs. 2.83A and B: CXR showing left apical arc-like calcification of the left ventricular aneurysm.

PLAIN FILM APPROACH TO CRITICAL CARE PATIENT WITH CXR FINDINGS OF PULMONARY CONGESTION/EDEMA (FIGS. 2.84, 2.85 AND TABLE 2.8)

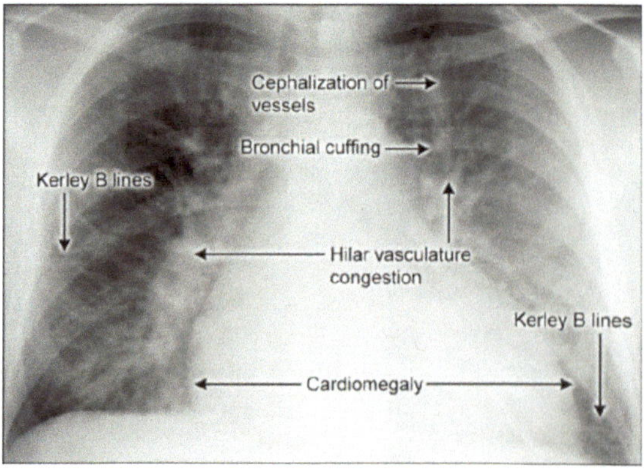

Fig. 2.84: CXR showing classical features of pulmonary edema.

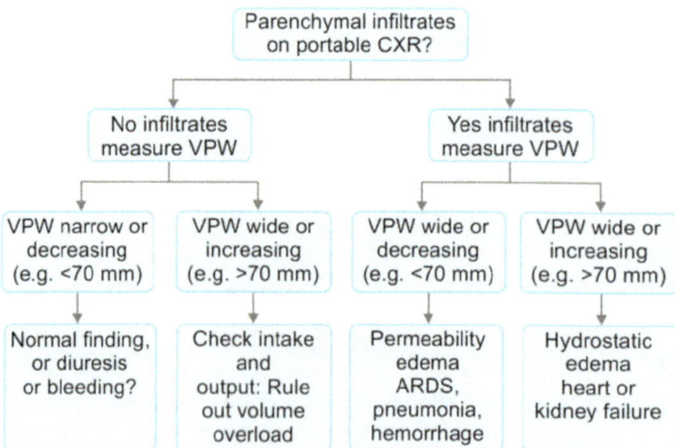

Fig. 2.85: Use of the vascular pedicle width from portable supine CXR.

TABLE 2.8: Differential diagnosis of different causes of pulmonary edema.

Radiological sign	***Cardiogenic***	***Renal***	***Capillary injury***
Heart shape	L-sided enlargement	R and L enlargement	Normal
Vascular pedicle width (SV)	+	++	Normal
Pulmonary blood distribution	Balanced or inverted	Balanced	Normal
Pulmonary blood volume	Normal or +	++	Normal
Septal lines	++	+	No
Peribronchial and vessel cuffing	+	+	No
Air bronchogram	+	+	++
Lung opacity distribution	Central and peripheral	Central	Peripheral and central
Pleural effusion	++	+	Uncommon
Soft-tissue chest wall	+	++	Normal

The VPW is measured by (1) Dropping a perpendicular line from the point at which the left subclavian artery exits the aortic arch and (2) Measuring across to the point at which the superior vena cava crosses the right mainstem bronchus **(Fig. 2.86)**.

Table 2.9 reflects left atrial pressure and its corresponding chest x-ray.

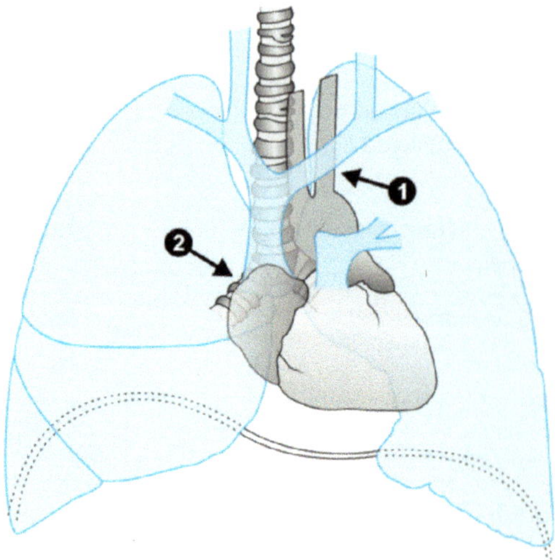

Fig. 2.86: Schematic diagram showing the site of measuring the vascular pedicle. Normal VPW range is 48 ± 5 mm.

TABLE 2.9: Left atrial pressure reflected on CXR.

Normal	*5–10 mm Hg*
Cephalization	10–15
Kerely B	15–20
Interstitial lung edema	20–25
Alveolar lung edema	> 25

Pericardial Effusion (Fig. 2.87)

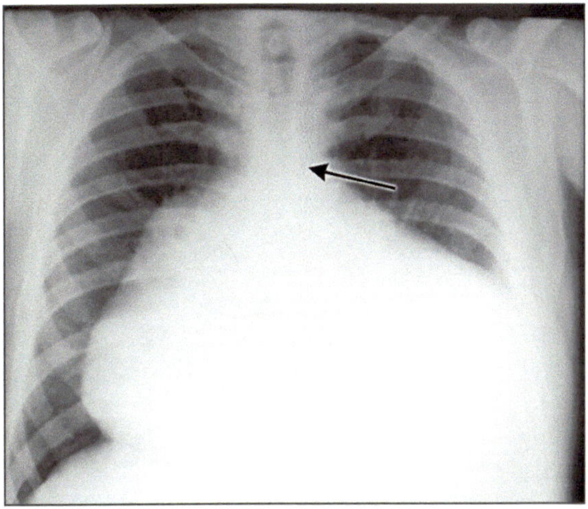

Fig. 2.87: CXR showing the classical appearance of enlarged heart with a narrow pedicle.

X-ray Signs of Pericardial Effusion

- Distinctness of the epicardial fat planes
- Normal pulmonary vasculature despite cardiomegaly
- Obliteration of retrosternal space
- Water bottle appearance of the enlarged cardiac silhouette
- Bilateral hilar overlay.

Pericardial Calcifications (Fig. 2.88)

- It is a consequence of tissue injury from inflammation, trauma causes include viral, tuberculosis, pyogenic infection.
- Incidence in patients with constructive pericarditis is 50 to 70%.

- The atrioventricular, interventricular groove and diaphragmatic border of the heart are common sites for calcification.
- The left atrium and left ventricle are usually spared.

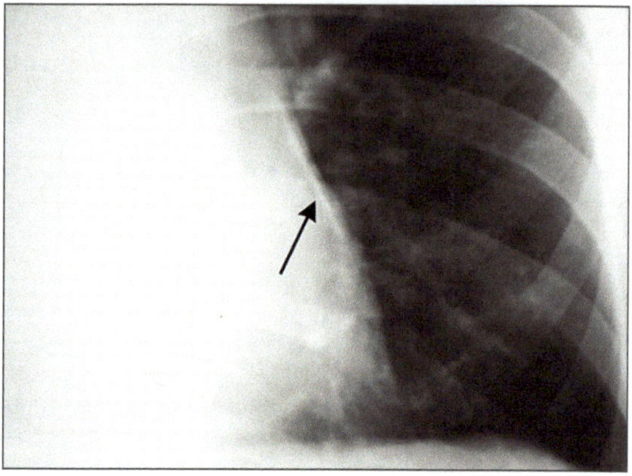

Fig. 2.88: CXR showing linear pericardial calcification.

MULTIPLE CHOICE QUESTIONS

1. **What is the most common cause of an enlarged cardiac silhouette on a chest X-ray?**
   a. Cardiomyopathy
   b. Pericardial effusion
   c. Left ventricular hypertrophy
   d. Pulmonary hypertension

2. **What is the classic radiographic finding in a patient with pneumothorax?**
   a. Butterfly pattern
   b. Flattened diaphragm
   c. Eggshell calcifications
   d. White-out lung

3. **Which imaging modality is most commonly used to diagnose pleural effusion?**
   a. Chest X-ray
   b. CT scan
   c. Ultrasound
   d. MRI

4. **Which of the following is not a common symptom of pleural effusion?**
   a. Dyspnea
   b. Chest pain
   c. Cough
   d. Hemoptysis

5. **What is the term used to describe pleural effusion with pus?**
   a. Serous effusion
   b. Transudative effusion
   c. Exudative effusion
   d. Empyema

6. **Which of the following is not a characteristic finding of pleural effusion on chest X-ray?**
   a. Blunting of costophrenic angles
   b. Meniscus sign
   c. Mediastinal shift
   d. Normal lung markings

7. **What is the primary treatment for pleural effusion?**
   a. Antibiotics
   b. Thoracentesis
   c. Corticosteroids
   d. Chemotherapy

8. **Which lung condition is typically associated with reduced lung volume on imaging studies?**
   a. Atelectasis
   b. Pneumonia
   c. Pulmonary embolism
   d. Bronchiectasis

9. **Which of the following is a common symptom of pneumonia but not typically associated with atelectasis?**
   a. Chest pain
   b. Cough with purulent sputum
   c. Dyspnea
   d. Hemoptysis

10. **Which lung condition is more likely to cause a shift of mediastinal structures towards the affected side on imaging?**
    a. Atelectasis
    b. Pneumonia
    c. Pleural effusion
    d. Pulmonary embolism

11. **What is the typical treatment approach for atelectasis?**
    a. Antibiotics
    b. Bronchodilators
    c. Chest physiotherapy
    d. Corticosteroids

12. **Which of the following is more commonly associated with a lobar pattern of lung involvement?**
    a. Atelectasis
    b. Pneumonia
    c. Pleural effusion
    d. Lung abscess

13. **What is a potential complication of untreated pneumonia but not typically seen in atelectasis?**
    a. Atelectasis of the contralateral lung
    b. Empyema
    c. Pulmonary fibrosis
    d. Pulmonary embolism

14. **Which condition is more likely to present with diffuse, patchy infiltrates on chest X-ray?**
    a. Atelectasis
    b. Pneumonia
    c. Pulmonary embolism
    d. Lung abscess

15. What is the main difference between transudate and exudate pleural effusion?

a. Transudate contains more protein
b. Exudate is caused by increased hydrostatic pressure
c. Exudate is caused by increased capillary permeability
d. Transudate is caused by inflammation

16. Which of the following conditions is more likely to cause transudate pleural effusion?

a. Congestive heart failure
b. Pneumonia
c. Tuberculosis
d. Lung cancer

17. Which laboratory finding is typically higher in exudate pleural effusion compared to transudate?

a. Total protein
b. Glucose
c. LDH (lactate dehydrogenase)
d. pH

18. What is the most common cause of exudate pleural effusion?

a. Congestive heart failure
b. Pulmonary embolism
c. Bacterial pneumonia
d. Hepatic cirrhosis

19. What is the primary cause of pleural plaque formation?

a. Smoking
b. Asbestos exposure
c. Viral infection
d. Genetic predisposition

20. Which of the following statements about pleural plaques is true?

a. They always progress to mesothelioma
b. They are typically symptomatic
c. They increase the risk of lung cancer
d. They are a common finding in pulmonary tuberculosis

21. Which of the following conditions presents with free air in the mediastinum on X-ray?
   a. Pneumomediastinum
   b. Morgagni hernia
   c. Heart border abnormalities
   d. Pulmonary embolism

22. Which of the following findings is characteristic of pulmonary arterial hypertension on chest X-ray?
   a. Enlarged pulmonary arteries
   b. Kerley B lines
   c. Pleural effusion
   d. Cardiomegaly

23. Which condition is associated with dilated central pulmonary arteries and a normal-sized heart on chest X-ray?
   a. Pulmonary arterial hypertension
   b. Pulmonary venous hypertension
   c. Pneumothorax
   d. Atelectasis

24. Which condition is characterized by redistribution of blood flow to the upper lung zones (cephalization) on chest X-ray?
   a. Pulmonary arterial hypertension
   b. Pulmonary venous hypertension
   c. Pulmonary embolism
   d. Pulmonary fibrosis

ANSWERS

1. c	2. b	3. c	4. d
5. d	6. d	7. b	8. a
9. b	10. a	11. c	12. b
13. b	14. b	15. c	16. a
17. c	18. c	19. b	20. c
21. a	22. a	23. a	24. b

CHAPTER 3

Disease Pattern

INTRODUCTION

- The chest radiograph is a composite image of the thoracic anatomy depicted in a gray scale based on the electron densities of the thoracic contents.
- The conspicuity of a region of interest is dependent on:
  - The region's attenuation of the X-ray beam
  - The additive attenuations of all structures anterior and posterior to it
  - The contrast between it, and its surrounding structures.

OPACITY

Opacities can be classified as:

- An opacity significantly denser than the heart
  - Calcium
  - Metal
  - Bone.
- An opacity equivalent or slightly denser than the heart
  - Water
  - Cells
  - Hemorrhage.

- An opacity not as dense as the heart—Hazy
  - Fat
  - Water
  - Cells
  - Hemorrhage.

Other Descriptions

- Shape
  - Linear **(Fig. 3.1)**
  - Tubular **(Fig. 3.2)**
  - Round **(Fig. 3.3)**.
- Borders
  - Smooth
  - Irregular/Shaggy **(Fig. 3.4)**.

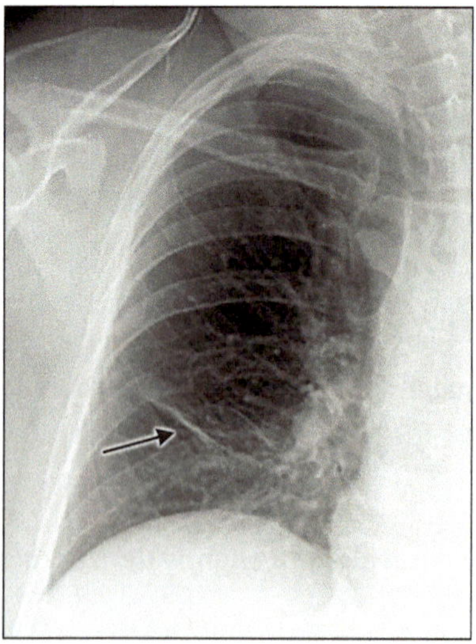

Fig. 3.1: A shadow resembling a line; hence, any elongated opacity of approximately uniform width—linear atelectasis.

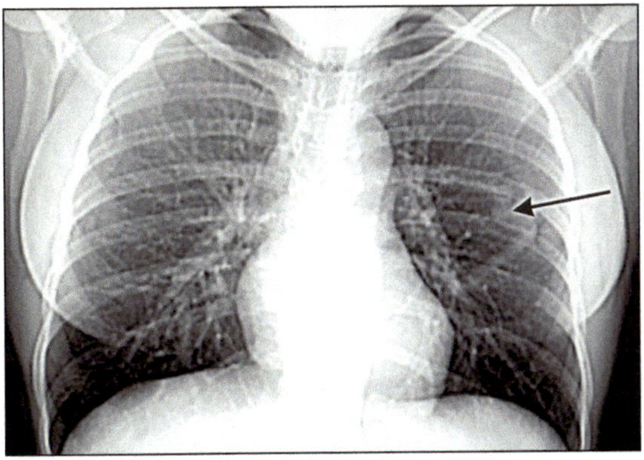

Fig. 3.2: Tubular opacity—pulmonary arteriovenous malformation.

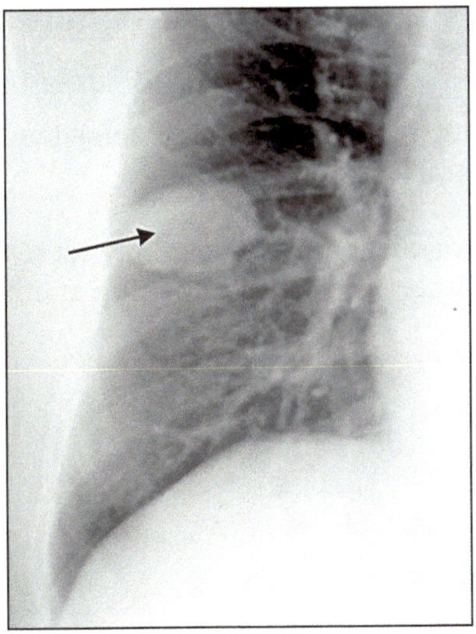

Fig. 3.3: Round opacity—pulmonary mass.

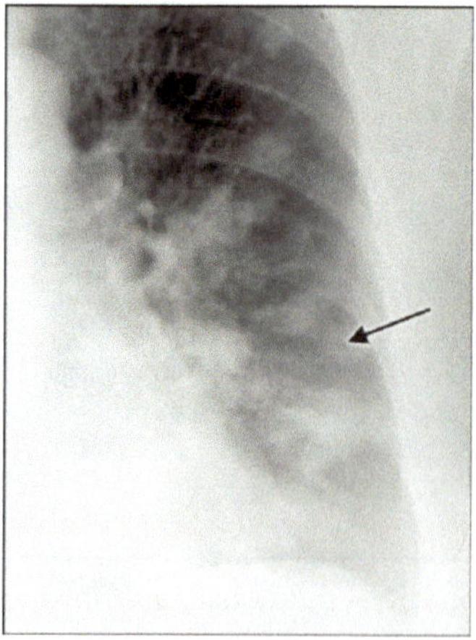

Fig. 3.4: Irregular opacity—metastasis.

Localized Opacity without Segmental Distribution

- Opacity with a uniform (homogenous) density
- Uni-/bilateral **(Figs. 3.6 and 3.7)**
- Focal rather than diffuse
- Air bronchogram is almost invariably present and should not be misinterpreted as examination of inhomogeneity.

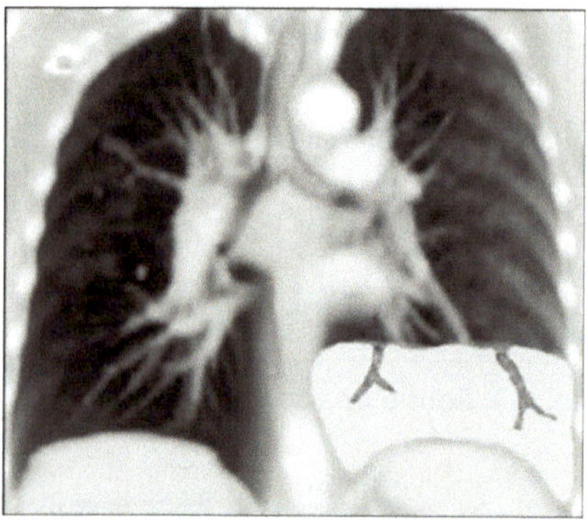

Fig. 3.5: Schematic diagram of consolidation.

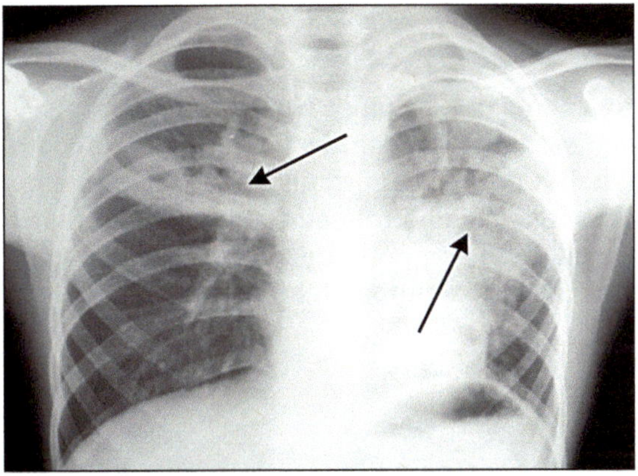

Fig. 3.6: CXR showing bilateral opacities with air bronchograms.

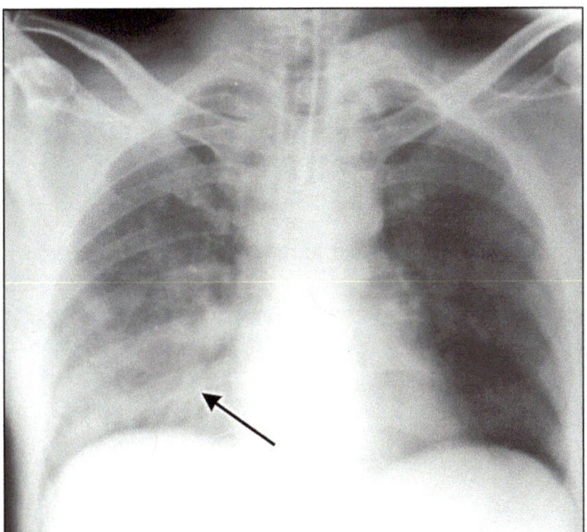

Fig. 3.7: CXR showing right lower lobe opacity.

Diffuse Disease with a Predominantly Reticular Pattern (See Figs. 3.8 and 3.9)

Thin linear opacities having a net-like appearance.

Opacities may be diffuse involving all lobes of both lungs, although they are often most marked in some regions.

The pattern may be related to such pathologic abnormalities as thickened interlobular septa, parenchymal cystic spaces, or interstitial fibrosis ("honeycombing").

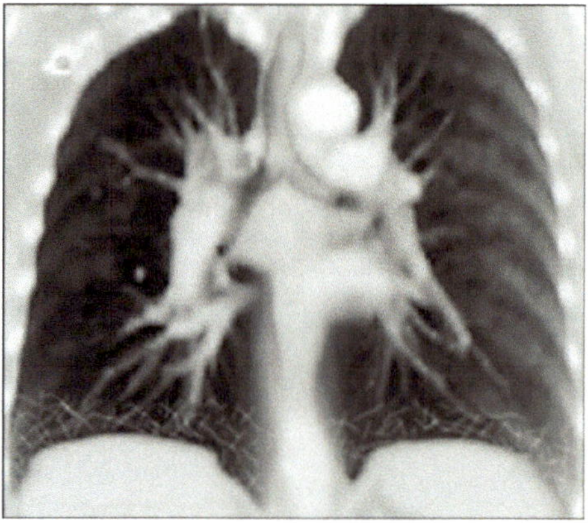

Fig. 3.8: Schematic diagram of reticular changes.

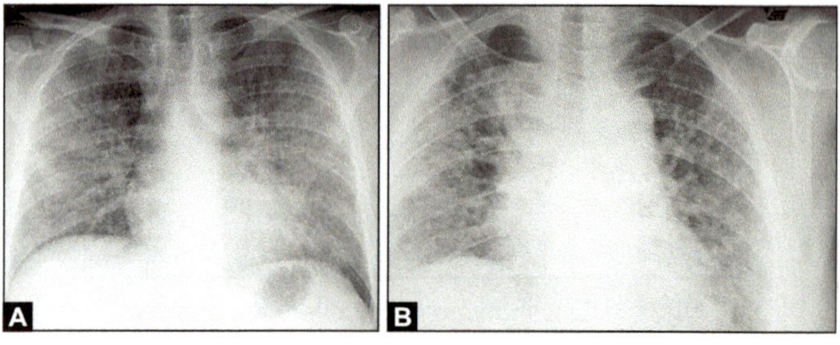

Figs. 3.9A and B: CXR in two different patients showing classical reticular opacities.

Diffuse Disease with a Predominantly Miliary Nodular Pattern (See Figs. 3.10 and 3.11A and B)

Diffuse nodular opacities typically measuring less than 5 mm in diameter.

The nodules may have well or poorly defined margins.

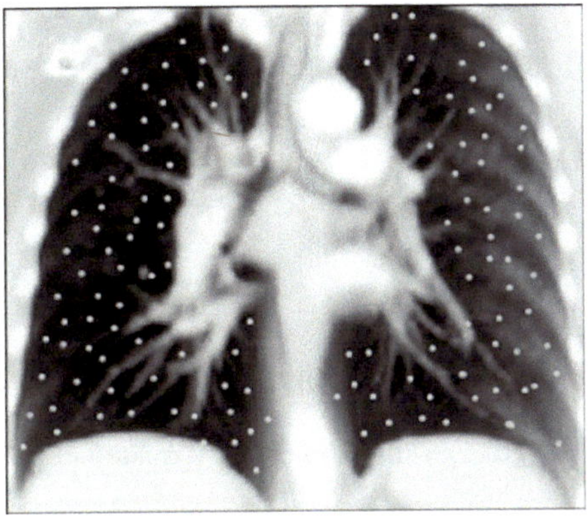

Fig. 3.10: Schematic diagram of nodules.

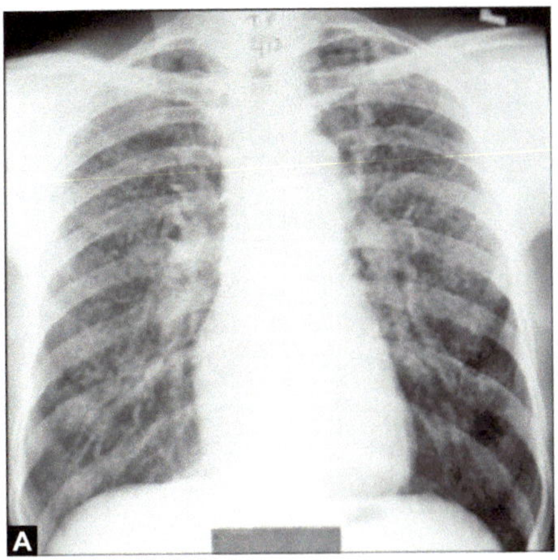

Fig. 3.11A

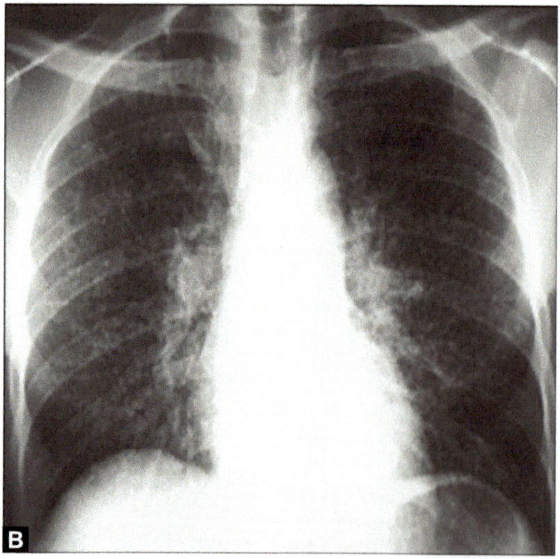

Figs. 3.11A and B: CXR showing classical miliary nodular pattern.

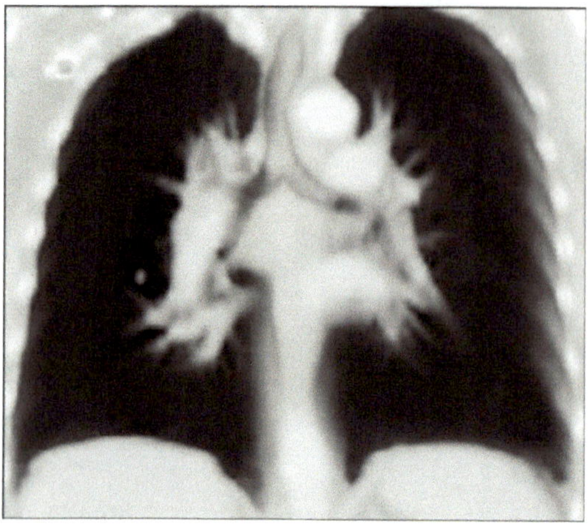

Fig. 3.12: Schematic diagram of diffuse translucency.

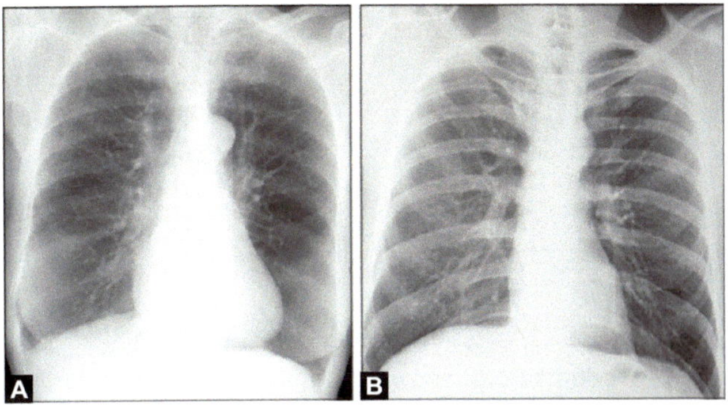

Figs. 3.13A and B: CXR in two different patients showing features of hyperinflation.

GENERALIZED PULMONARY TRANSLUCENCY (FIGS. 3.12 TO 3.16)

Diffuse hyperlucency of the lungs associated with a splaying of the pulmonary vascular bundle **(Figs. 3.12 and 3.13)**.

Unilateral, Lobar, or Segmental Pulmonary Hyperlucency (Figs. 3.14 to 3.16)

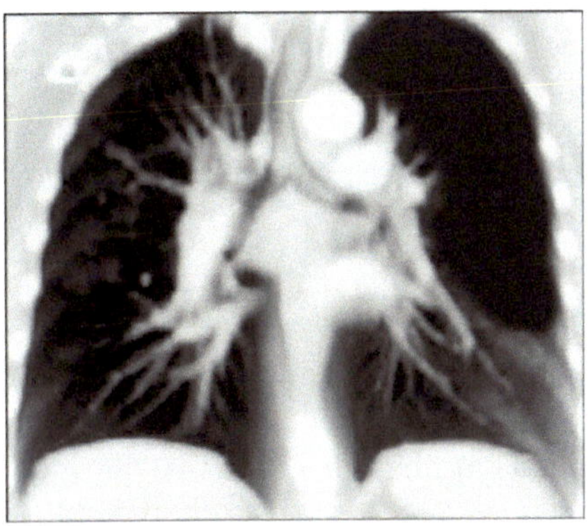

Fig. 3.14: Schematic diagram of focal translucency.

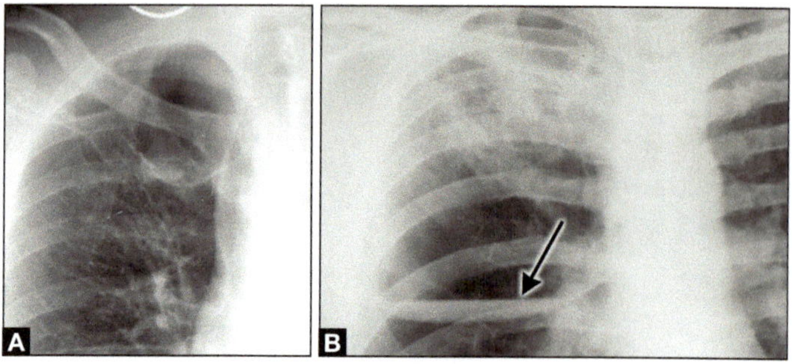

Figs. 3.15A and B: CXR showing right upper lobe bulla in two different patients. In Figure B note the air fluid level indicating infection (arrow).

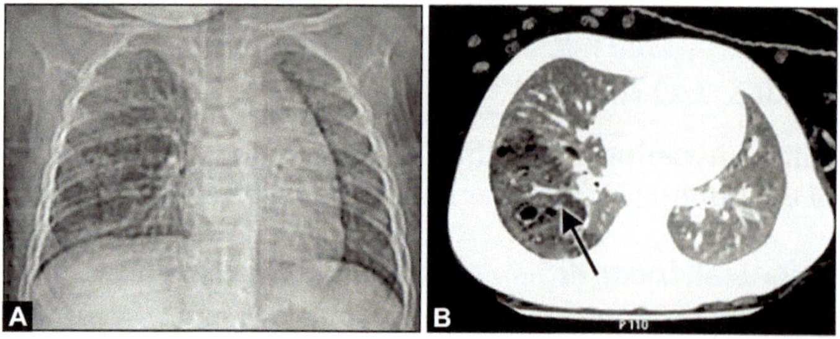

Figs. 3.16A and B: Digital scanogram and axial HRCT showing a right lower lobe lucency with multiple cysts suggestive of congenital cystadenamatoid malformation (arrow).

Hilar and Mediastinal Lymph Node Enlargement (Figs. 3.17 to 3.19)

- Expanded often lobulated hilar region
- Uni-/bilateral
- Mediastinal disease most often manifested as enlargement of right paratracheal, subcarinal, aortopulmonary or paraspinal lymph nodes.

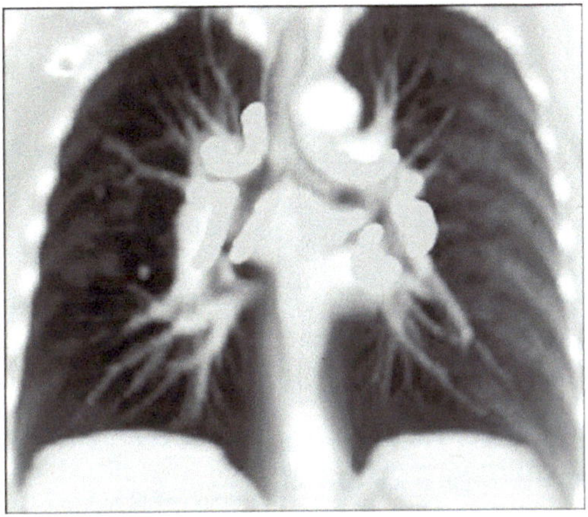

Fig. 3.17: Schematic diagram of nodes.

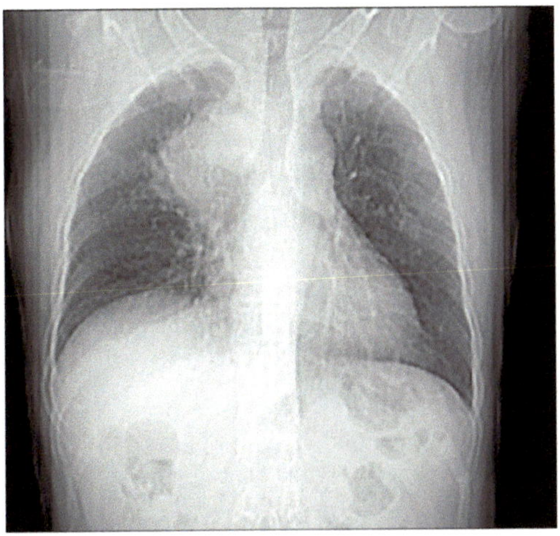

Fig. 3.18: CXR showing a large right paratracheal node.

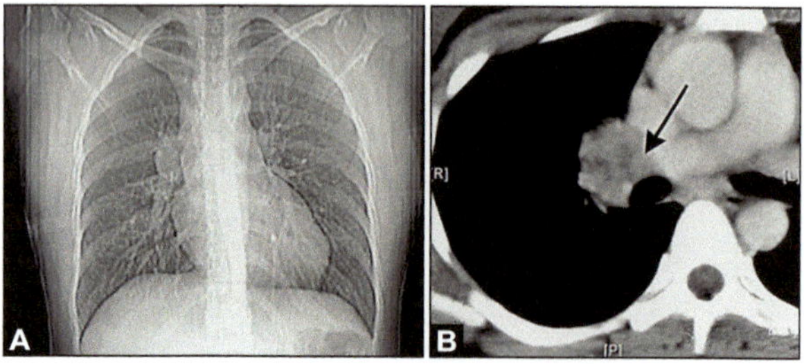

Figs. 3.19A and B: Digital scanogram and axial CECT showing right hilar node (arrow).

Masses Situated Predominantly in Anterior Mediastinal Compartment (Figs. 3.20 to 3.23)

- Anterior mediastinum is bounded anteriorly by the sternum.

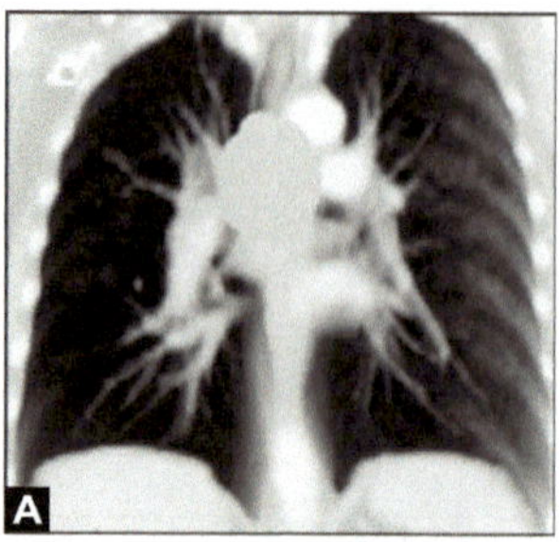

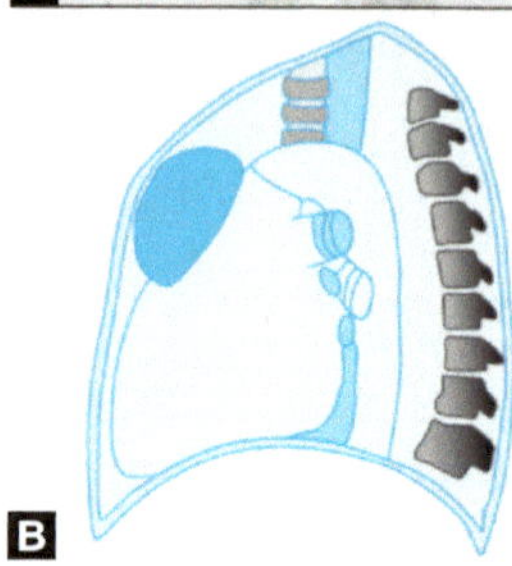

Figs. 3.20A and B: Schematic diagram of anterior mediastinum.

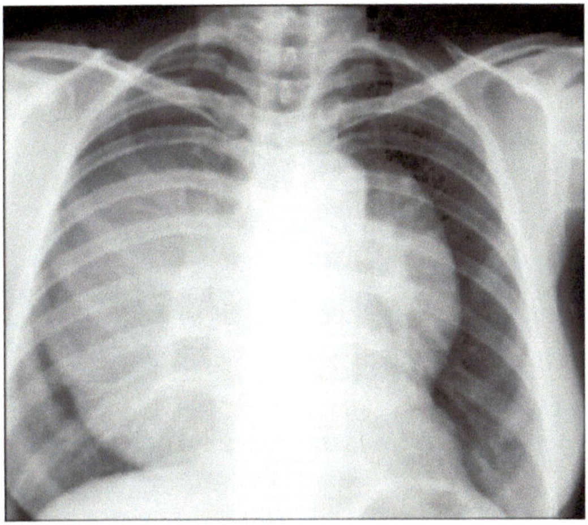

Fig. 3.21: CXR showing large well-marginated opacity through which the right hilum is well seen (case of anterior mediastinal cyst).

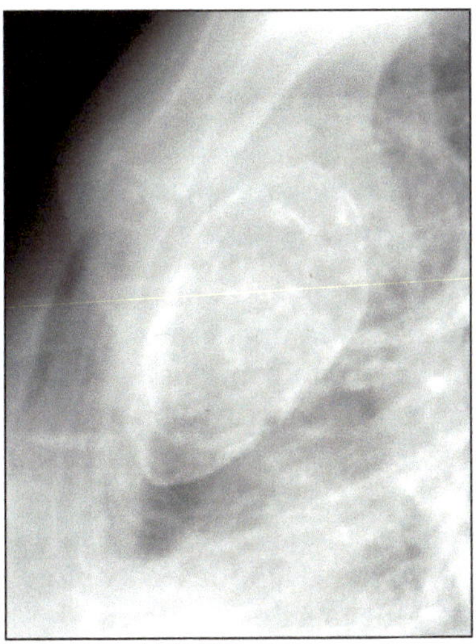

Fig. 3.22: Lateral X-ray showing a well-marginated calcified mass in the anterior mediastinum.

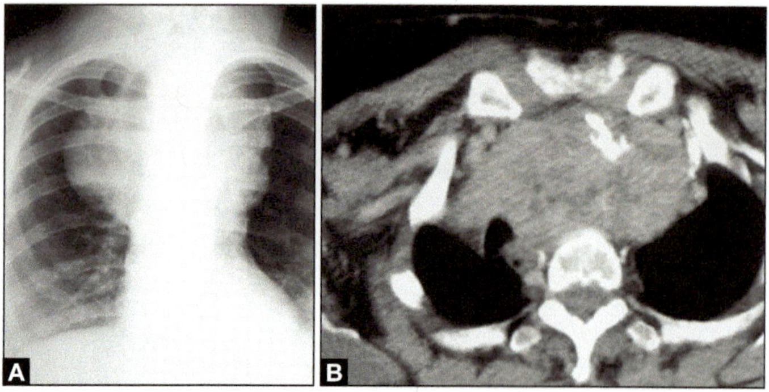

Figs. 3.23A and B: CXR and axial CT section showing a large heterogenous mass in the superior and anterior mediastinum—case of large retrosternal goiter.

- Posteriorly by the pericardium, aorta, and brachiocephalic vessels.

For practical reasons, a mass is considered to lie in the anterior compartment when it is situated in the region anterior to a line drawn along the anterior border of the trachea and the posterior border of the heart.

Masses Situated Predominantly in Middle and Posterior Mediastinal Compartments (Figs. 3.23 to 3.27)

Middle mediastinum contains → heart, major vessels, trachea and main bronchi, lymph nodes, phrenic and vagus nerves.

Posterior mediastinum contains → descending thoracic aorta, esophagus, thoracic duct, vagus nerves and lymph nodes.

On lateral CXR, these 2 compartments are considered together.

- Lesion can be considered to lie in the middle or posterior compartment when it is located below a line drawn through anterior aspect of trachea and posterior aspect of heart and the line drawn through the anterior margins of vertebral bodies.

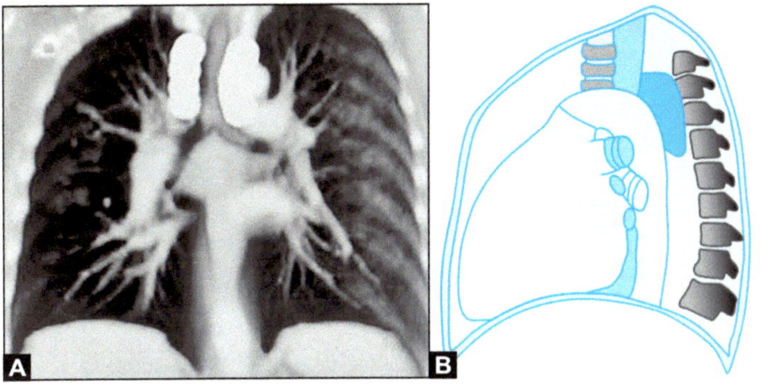

Figs. 3.24A and B: Schematic diagram of middle and posterior mediastinum.

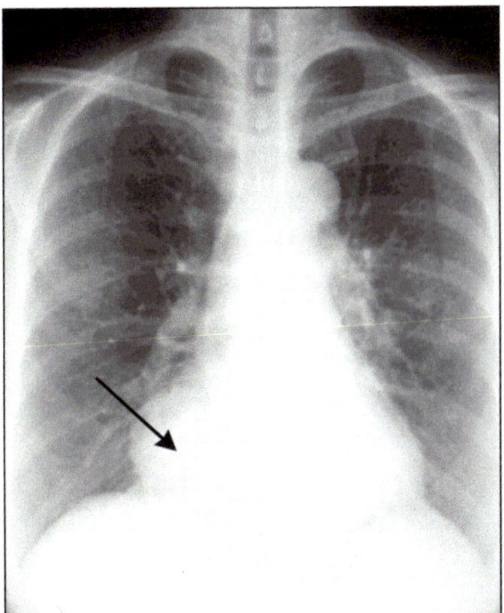

Fig. 3.25: CXR showing a right cardiophrenic angle opacity—case of pericardial cyst (arrow).

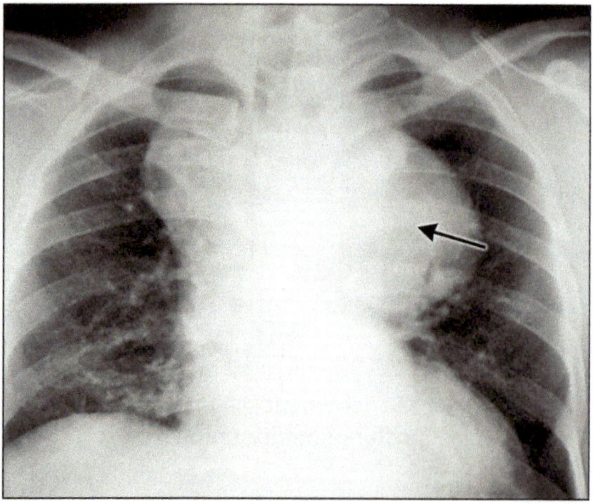

Fig. 3.26: CXR showing a lobulated opacity (arrow) causing widening of mediastinum—case of aortic arch aneurysm.

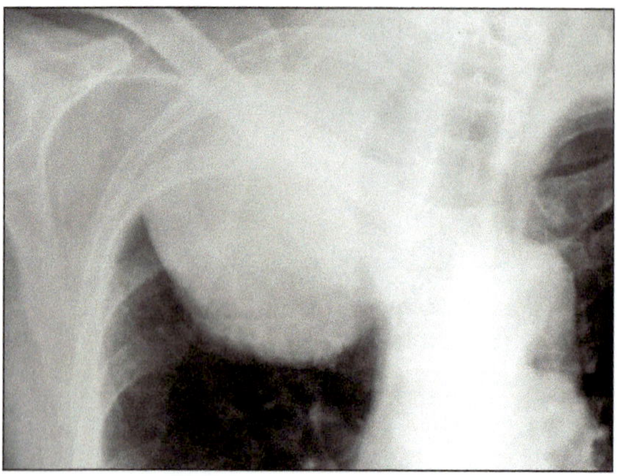

Fig. 3.27: CXR showing a well-marginated right upper zone opacity (case of neural tumor).

Masses Situated in the Paravertebral Region (Fig. 3.28)

Posterior limit of mediastinum is formed by the anterior surface of the vertebral column.

On lateral CXR, a mass can be considered to be in the paravertebral region when it lies posterior to the anterior surface of vertebral bodies.

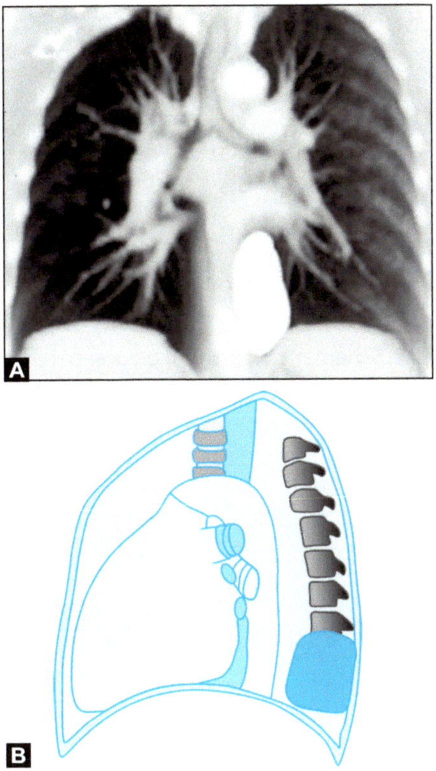

Figs. 3.28A and B: Schematic diagram of paravertebral lesions.

LOCALIZED PLEURAL BASED/CHEST WALL OPACITY (SEE FIGS. 3.29 AND 3.30)

Peripheral mass with obtuse margins that abuts the chest wall and pleura with or without rib destruction.

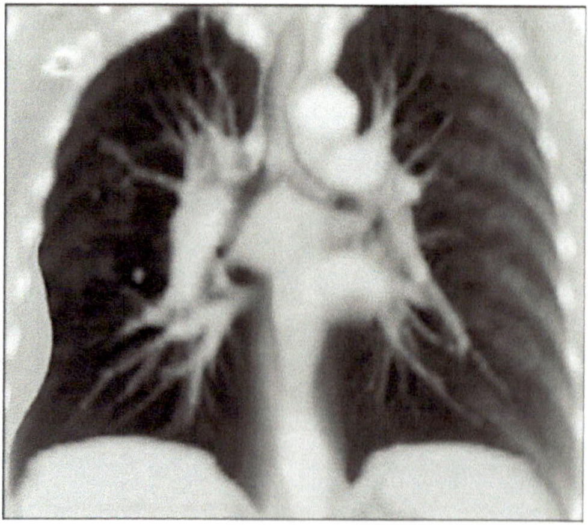

Fig. 3.29: Schematic diagram of pleural based lesion.

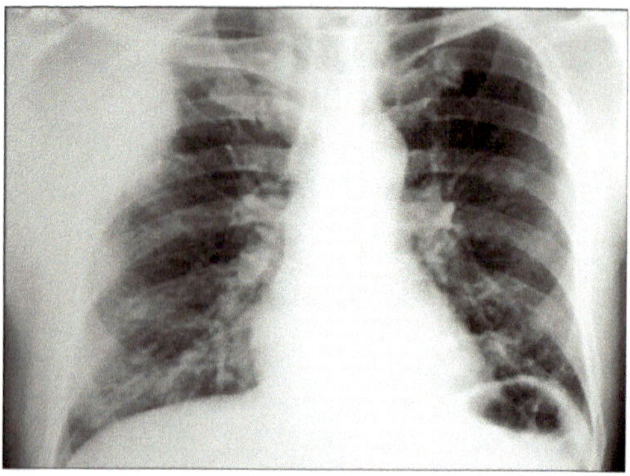

Fig. 3.30: CXR showing right upper zone pleural based soft tissue mass.

Diffuse Pleural Thickening (Figs. 3.31 to 3.33)

Diffuse in this context is defined as an uninterrupted pleural opacity extending over at least 1/4th of the chest wall with or without obliteration of the costophrenic sulcus.

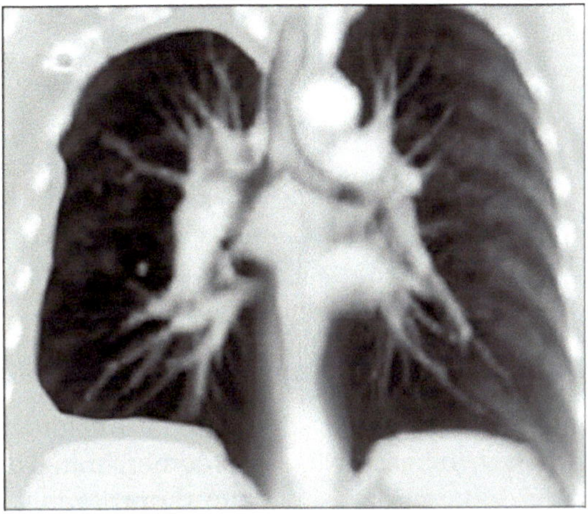

Fig. 3.31: Schematic diagram of pleural thickening.

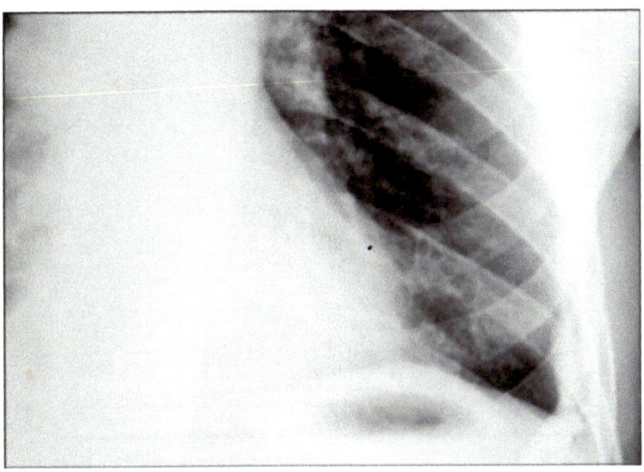

Fig. 3.32: CXR showing left lateral and basal pleural thickening.

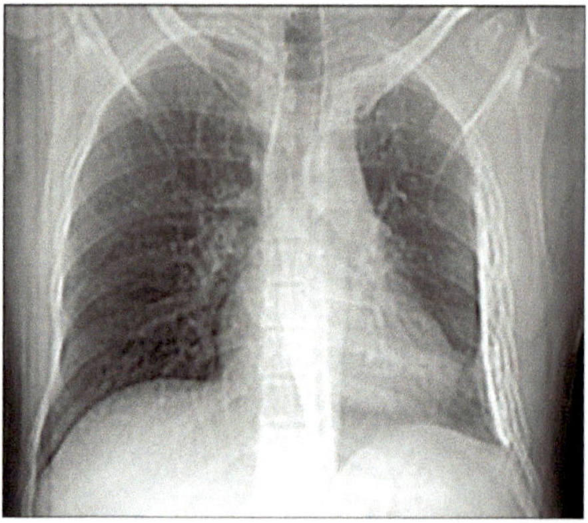

Fig. 3.33: Digital scanogram showing left pleural diffuse thickening with calcification.

PLEURAL EFFUSION WITH LARGE CARDIAC SILHOUETTE

Enlargement of the cardiac silhouette is considered to be present when an increase in its size is demonstrated on serial radiographs or the cardiac silhouette-thorax ratio is greater than 1:2 (50%) **(Figs. 3.34 and 3.35)**.

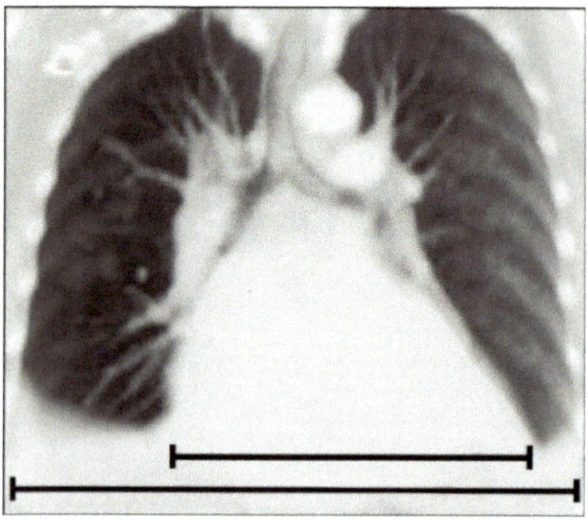

Fig. 3.34: Schematic diagram of CTR.

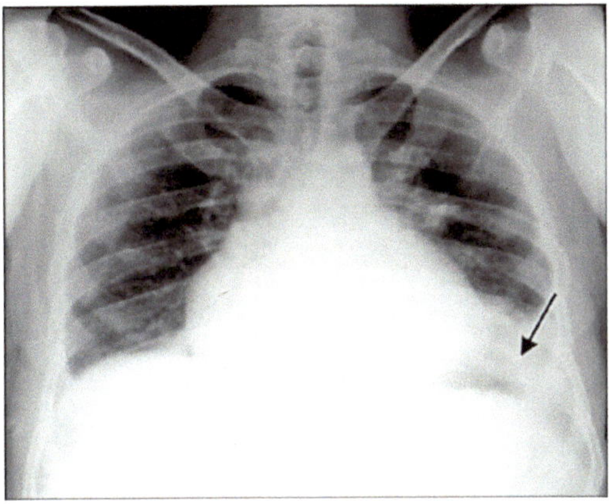

Fig. 3.35: CXR showing enlarged heart with bilateral pleural effusion more evident on the left side.

Pleural Effusion without Pulmonary Disease (Figs. 3.36 and 3.37)

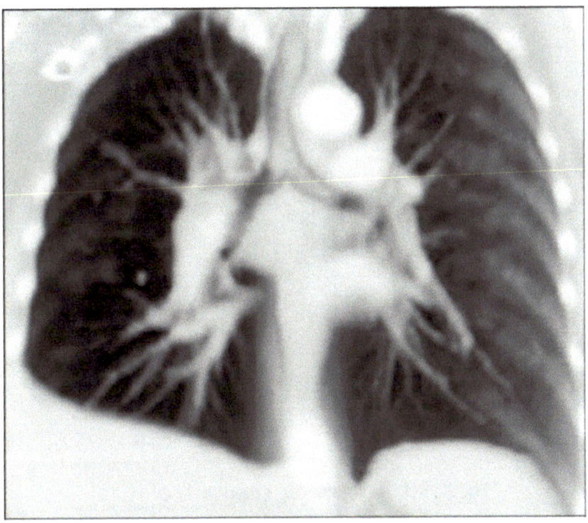

Fig. 3.36: Schematic diagram of pleuroparenchymal disease.

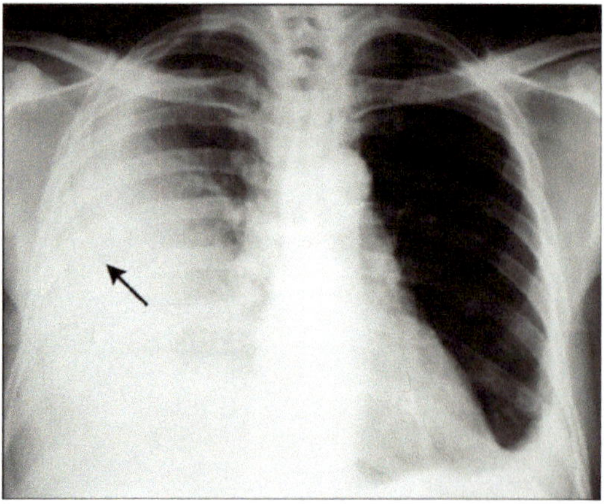

Fig. 3.37: CXR showing bilateral pleural effusion more evident on the right side.

Pleural Effusion with Pulmonary Disease (Figs. 3.38 to 3.40)

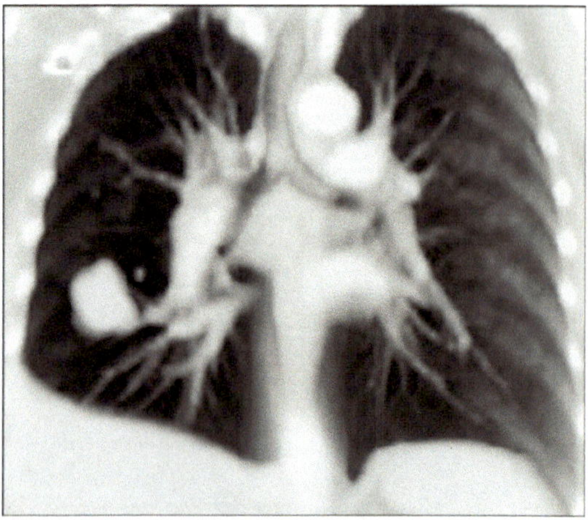

Fig. 3.38: Schematic diagram of focal parenchymal and pleural disease.

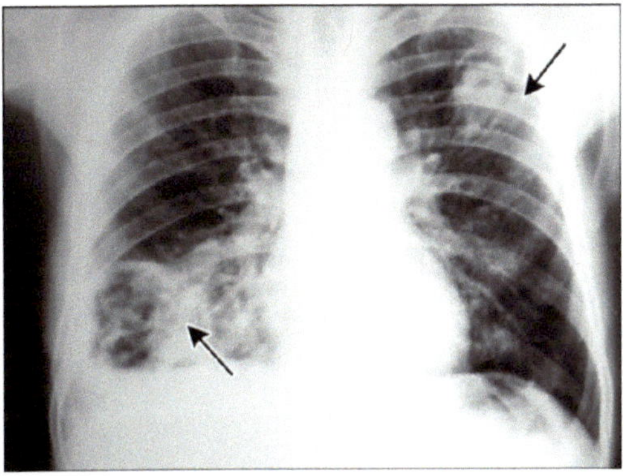

Fig. 3.39: CXR showing right lower zone pneumonitis with pleural effusion. Note the left upper lobe fungal ball.

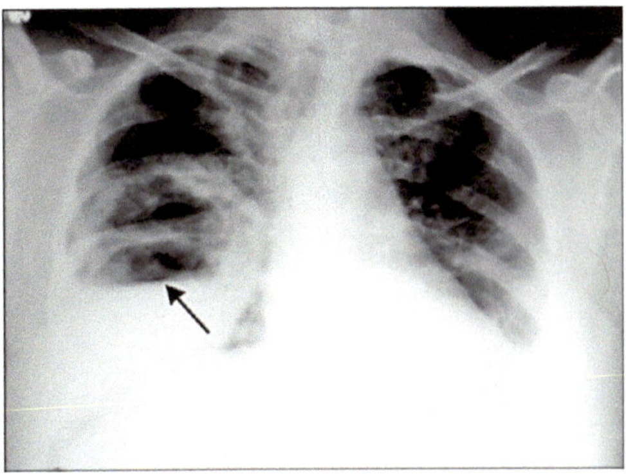

Fig. 3.40: CXR showing right lower lobe abscess with pleural effusion. Note the air fluid level (arrow).

LOCALIZED OPACITY WITH SEGMENTAL DISTRIBUTION (FIGS. 3.41 TO 3.43)

An opacity with a uniform (homogeneous) density located in the site of one or more bronchopulmonary segments. Masses of infective pneumonia can cause this appearance.

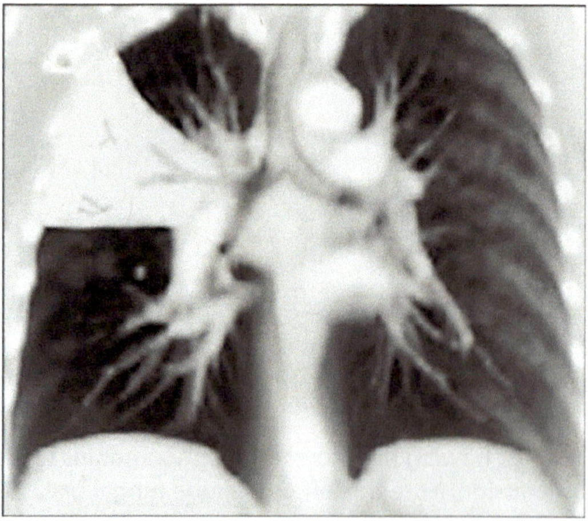

Fig. 3.41: Schematic diagram of segmental opacity.

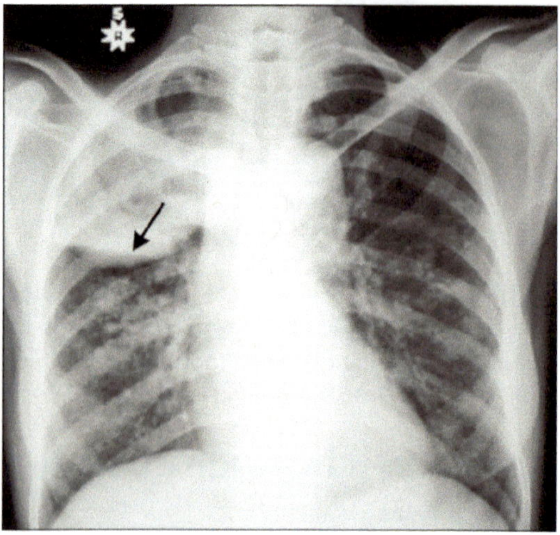

Fig. 3.42: CXR showing right upper lobe mass causing fissural bulging (arrow).

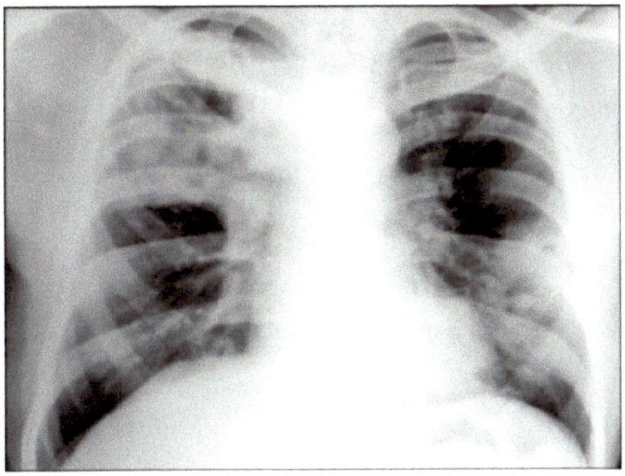

Fig. 3.43: CXR showing right upper and left lobe consolidations.

CYSTIC AND CAVITARY DISEASE (FIGS. 3.44 TO 3.49)

- This pattern includes all forms of pulmonary disease characterized by one or several circumscribed air-containing spaces, each of which is bordered by distinct walls, including cavitated pneumonia or carcinoma, and cystic bronchiectasis.

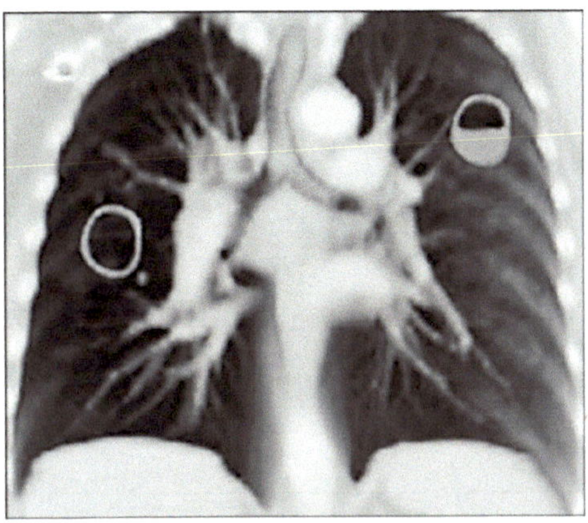

Fig. 3.44: Schematic diagram of cavitary lesion.

- An air-fluid level may or may not be present.
- Cavities may be single or multiple.

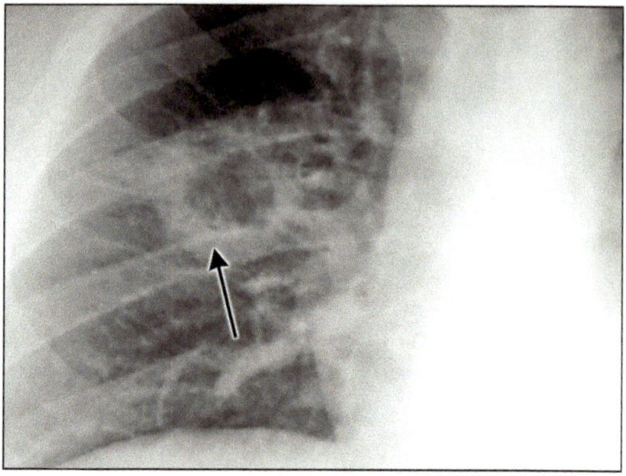

Fig. 3.45: CXR showing right mid-zone thick-walled cavity with adjacent satellite lesions suggestive of abscess.

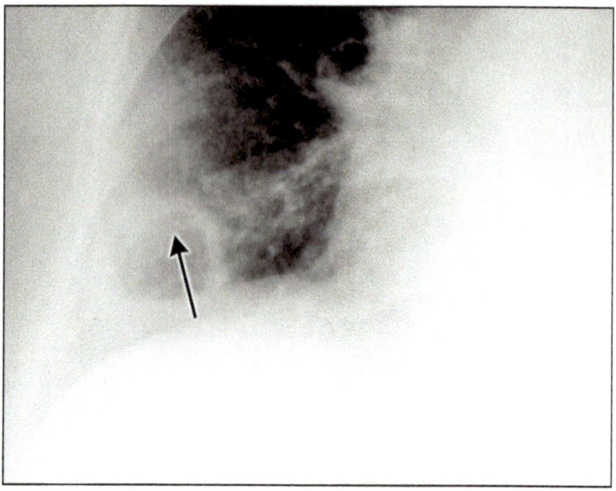

Fig. 3.46: CXR showing right lower zone costophrenic angle cavity with fluid level (arrow).

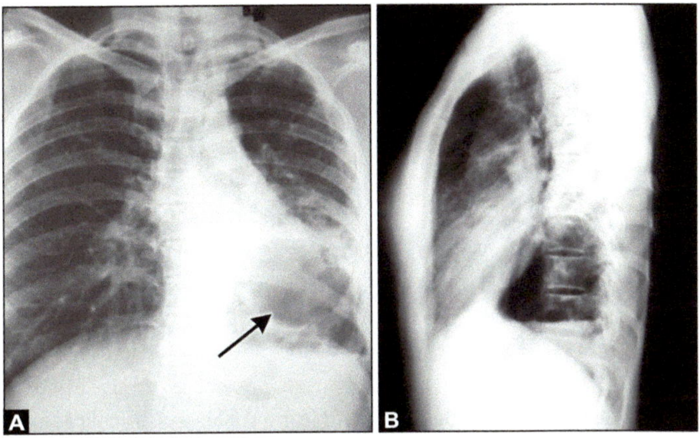

Figs. 3.47A and B: CXR PA and lateral view showing a large cyst with air fluid level and uniform thick walls.

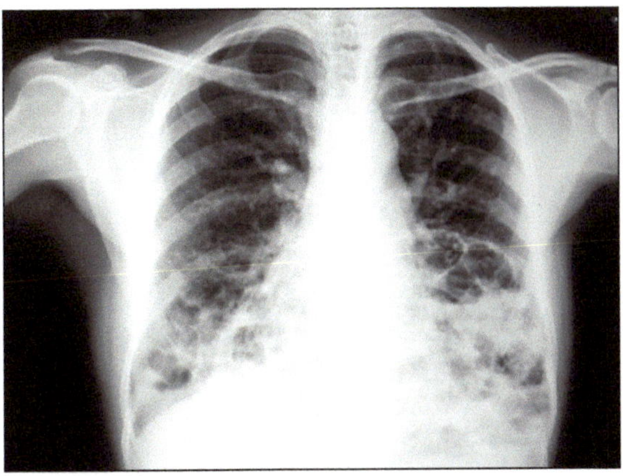

Fig. 3.48: CXR showing bilateral lower lobe conglomerate cyst with few cysts showing fluid levels—case of infected bronchiectasis.

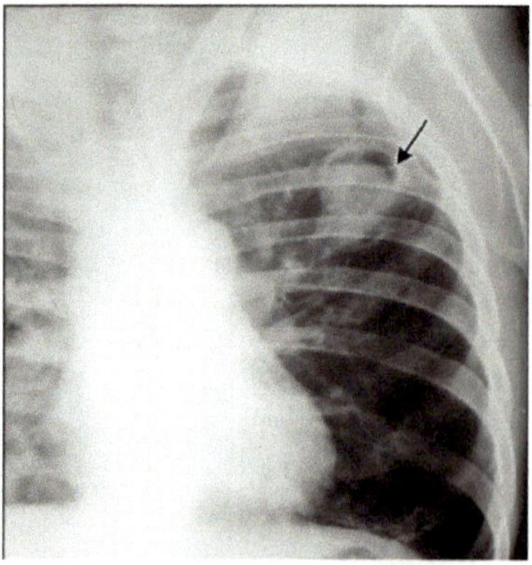

Fig. 3.49: Left upper lobe cavity with fungal ball—classical case of air crescent sign of fungal ball.

Solitary Pulmonary Mass (Figs. 3.50 to 3.52)

A discrete opacity >3 cm in diameter.

It may have any contour (smooth, lobulated, or umbilicated). May or may not be calcified.

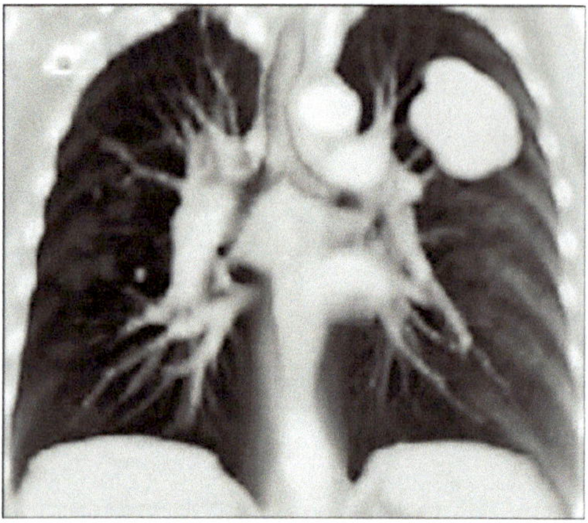

Fig. 3.50: Schematic diagram of focal mass.

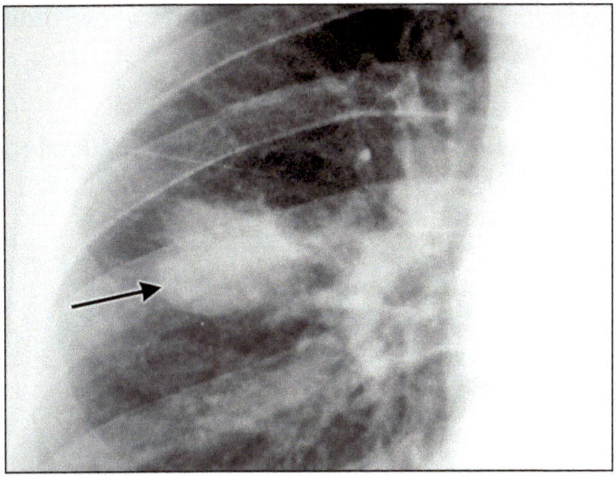

Fig. 3.51: CXR showing right mid zone opacity.

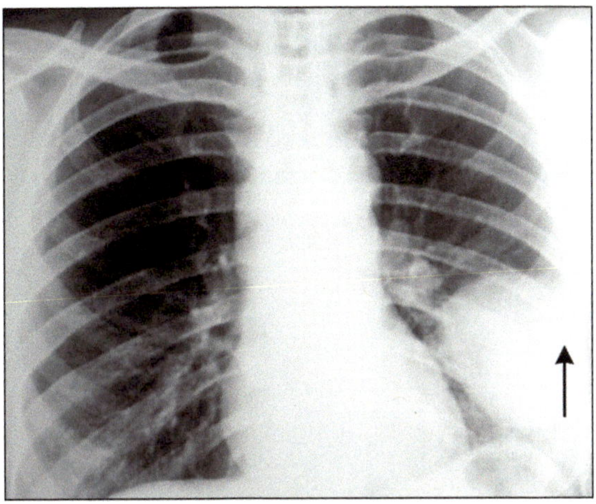

Fig. 3.52: CXR showing left lower lobe soft tissue opacity.

Multiple Pulmonary Nodules or Masses, with or without Cavitation (Figs. 3.53 to 3.56)

- Multiple opacities > 5 mm in diameter
- They may have any contour (smooth, lobulated, or umbilicated)
- May or may not be calcified.

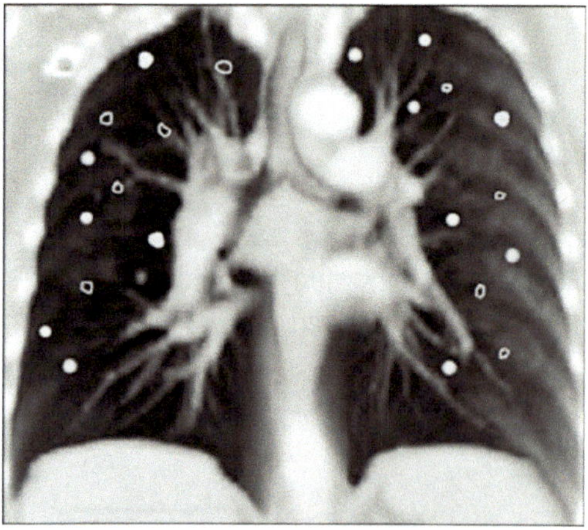

Fig. 3.53: Schematic diagram of multiple nodules.

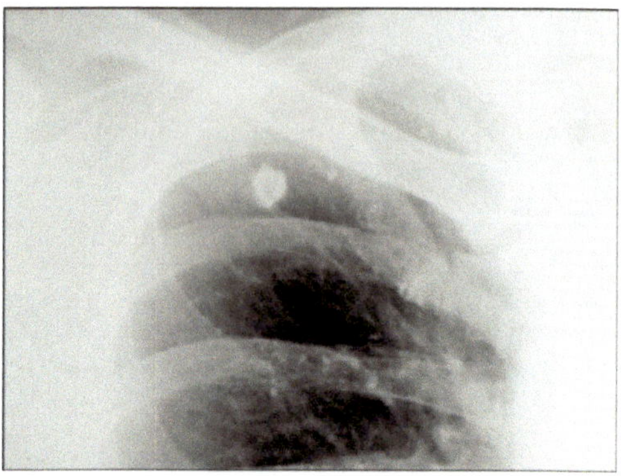

Fig. 3.54: CXR showing right upper lobe calcified nodule.

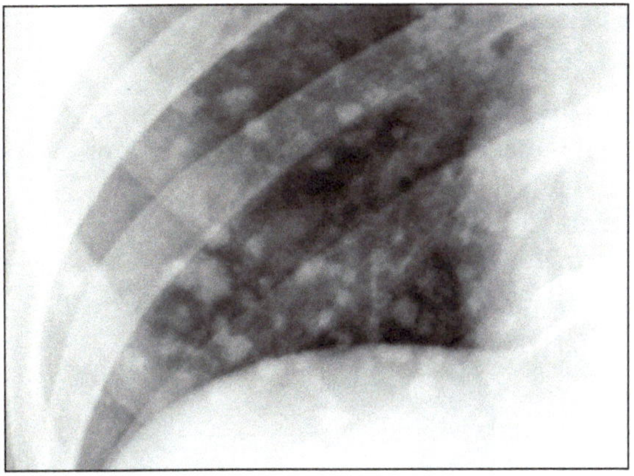

Fig. 3.55: CXR showing right mid and lower zone multiple calcified nodules.

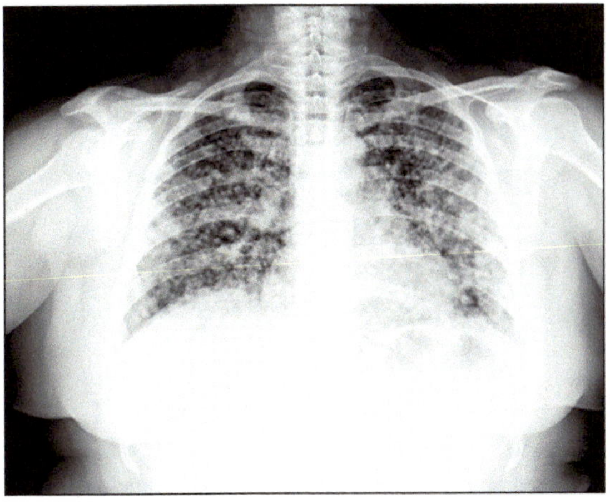

Fig. 3.56: CXR showing bilateral multiple lung nodules—typical features of metastasis.

Diffuse Disease with a Predominantly Air-Space Pattern (Figs 3.57 to 3.60)

Opacities involving several lobes of both lungs.
Though the disease is widespread, it does not necessarily affect all lung regions uniformly.

For example, lower lung zones may be involved to a greater or lesser degree than the upper.

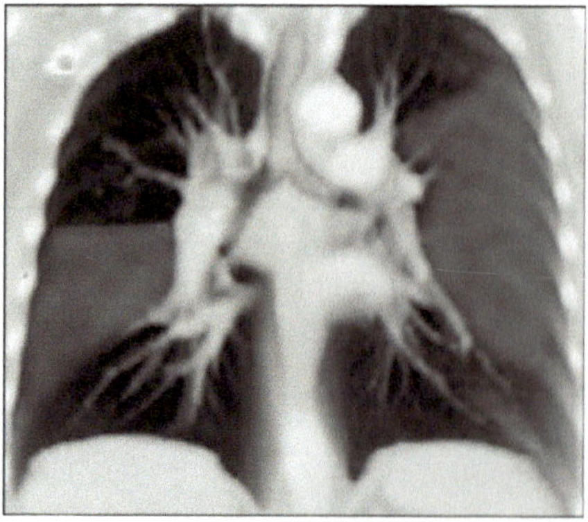

Fig. 3.57: Schematic diagram of airspace disease.

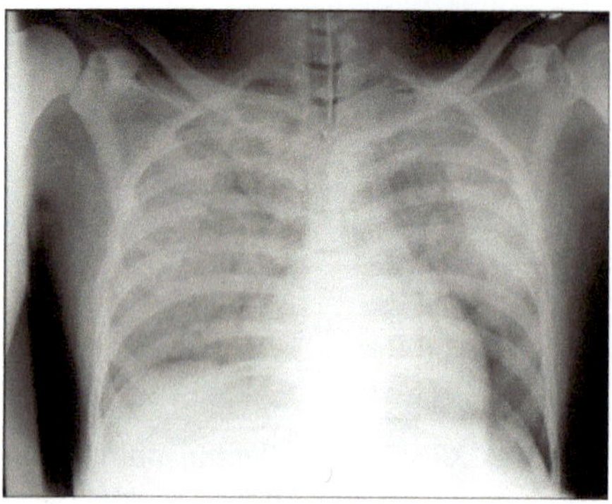

Fig. 3.58: ARDS CXR in a patient with history of toxic gas inhalation showing bilateral diffuse parenchymal opacities.

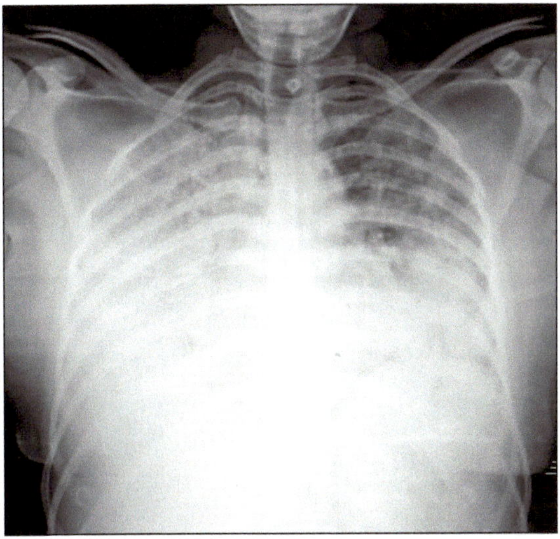

Fig. 3.59: CXR showing diffuse parenchymal opacity in a patient with acute interstitial pneumonia.

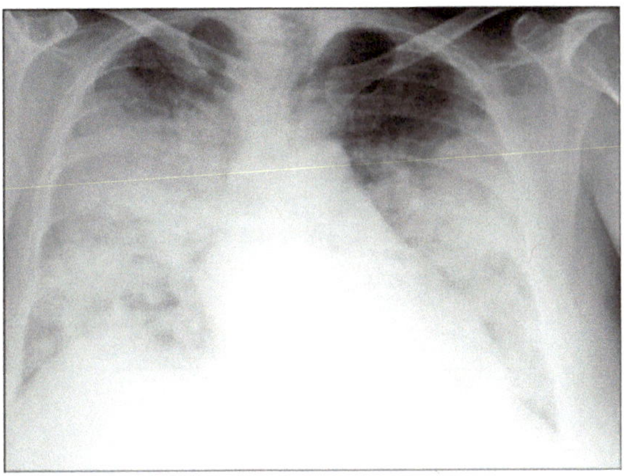

Fig. 3.60: Pulmonary edema with classical bat's wing appearance.

FIBROCAVITARY DISEASE (FIGS. 3.61 TO 3.65)

Patterns of Tuberculosis

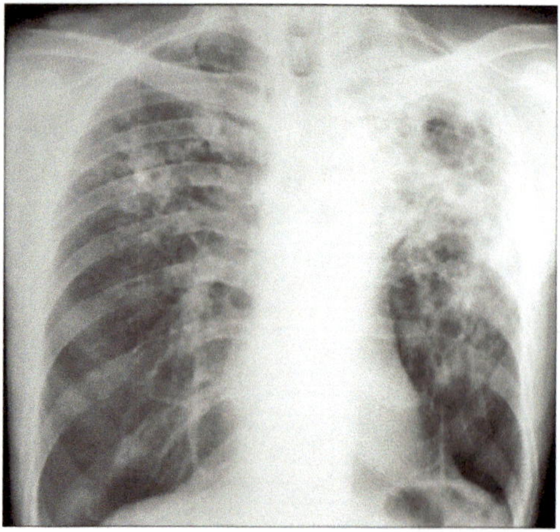

Fig. 3.61: CXR showing bilateral upper lobe fibrocavitary disease, more evident on the left side.

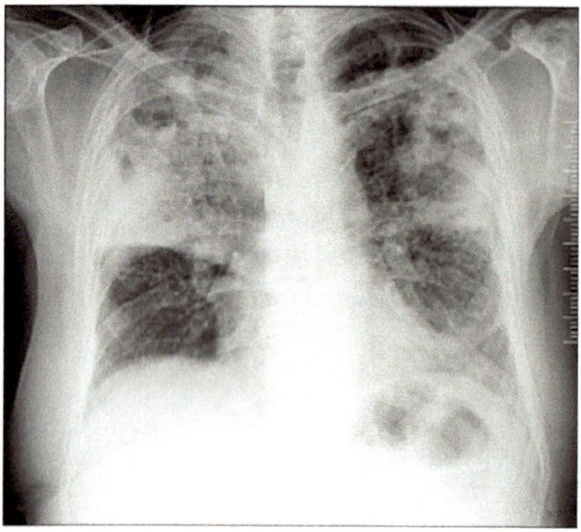

Fig. 3.62: CXR showing bilateral upper lobe cavitary consolidation.

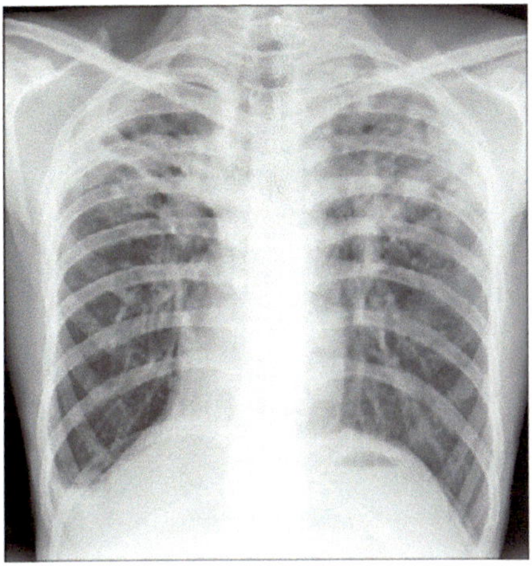

Fig. 3.63: CXR showing bilateral upper lobe fibrosis with sequelae.

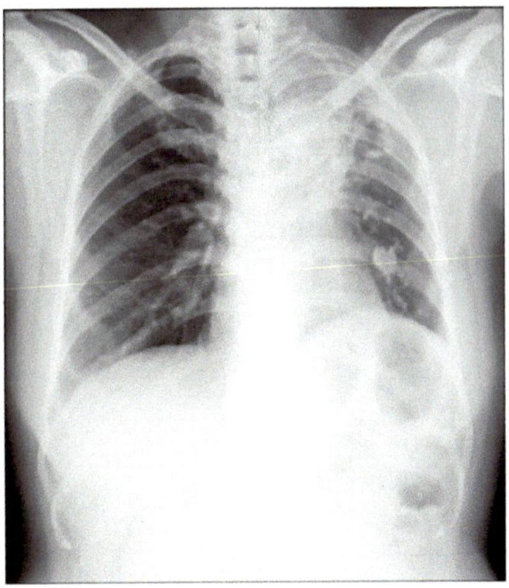

Fig. 3.64: CXR showing left upper lobe fibrosis with collapse. Note the elevated left hemidiaphragm.

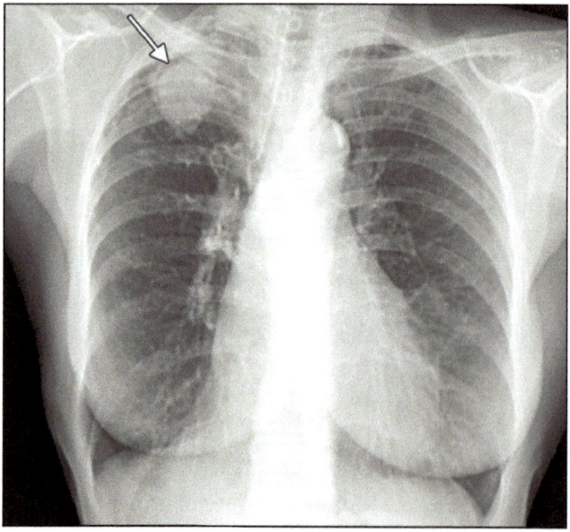

Fig. 3.65: CXR showing right upper lobe cavity with fungal ball. Note the Monod sign (air crescent).

COMMON TUBES AND LINES IN ICU

Radiographic monitoring of various devices used in postoperative and ill patients is essential to reduce the incidence of iatrogenic and associated complications. Basic knowledge regarding their normal positioning is useful.

Central Venous Line and Tracheostomy Tube

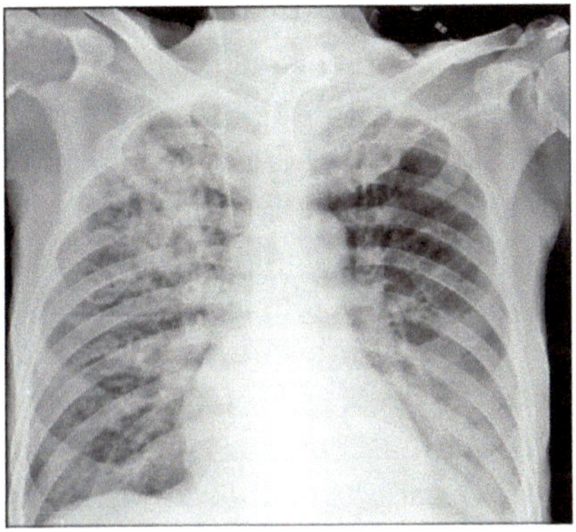

Fig. 3.66: CXR AP view in an ICU patient showing right central venous line and tracheostomy tube 3–5 cm above carina.

TRACHEOSTOMY (FIGS. 3.66 AND 3.67)

A well placed position will be parallel to the long axis of trachea, approximately one-third to two-thirds the diameter of trachea and positioned several cm from the carina.

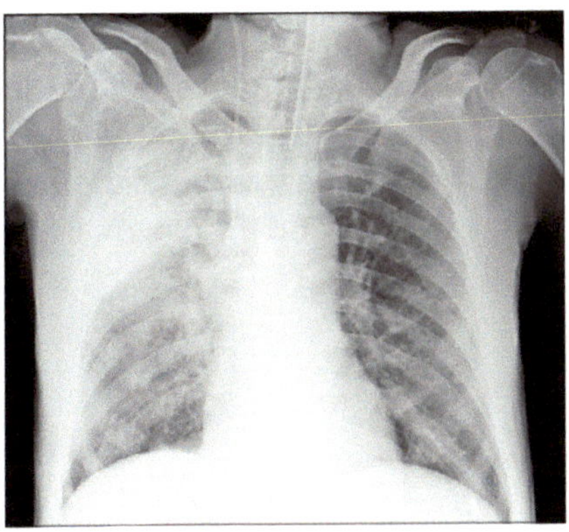

Fig. 3.67: CXR AP view showing central venous line and endotracheal tube.

CENTRAL VENOUS LINE (FIG. 3.66)

Positioning of a central venous line is a common reason for requesting a CXR. For correct positioning, the tip of the line should be located within the superior vena cava (SVC) approximately at the level of the carina. This approximates the level of the pericardial reflection and just below where the left and right brachiocephalic veins enter the SVC. The depth to which this is placed "at skin" from a mid- or low-right internal jugular approach can be calculated in adults by a modification of Peres' formula: Depth = patient's height in cm/10 minus 2 cm. For left sided lines normally add roughly 3 cm in adults to allow for the course through the left brachiocephalic vein.

ENDOTRACHEAL TUBE

Endotracheal tube (ETT): Safe distance is 5 cm from carina, at the level of the clavicles in infants. This distance is needed to ensure that it does not descend into the right main stem bronchus, with flexion of head and does not ascend to pharynx on extension.

Dees method for carina—this involves defining the aortic arch and then drawing a line inferomedially through the middle of the arch at a 45 degree angle to the midline. The intersection of the midline and the diagonal line is the most likely position of the carina.

PACEMAKER (FIG. 3.68)

Tip should be at the apex of the heart with no angulation along the length on lateral view it should point anteriorly and be located deep to the epicardial fat stripe. The wire should be checked at two stress points as it passes through the chest wall, and the myocardial anchor.

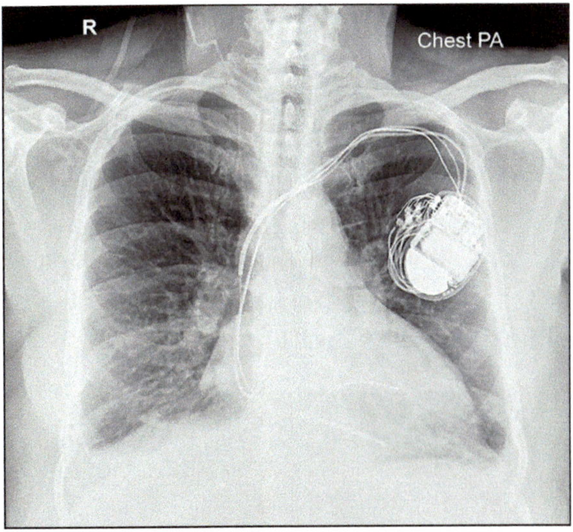

Fig. 3.68: CXR AP view showing pacemaker with the leads.

THORACOSTOMY TUBE (FIG. 3.69)

In order for thoracostomy tubes to function properly all of the fenestrations in the tube must be within the thoracic cavity. The last side-hole in a thoracostomy tube is indicated by a gap in the radiopaque line. If this interruption in the radiopaque line is not within the thoracic cavity or there is evidence of subcutaneous air, then the tube may not have been completely inserted.

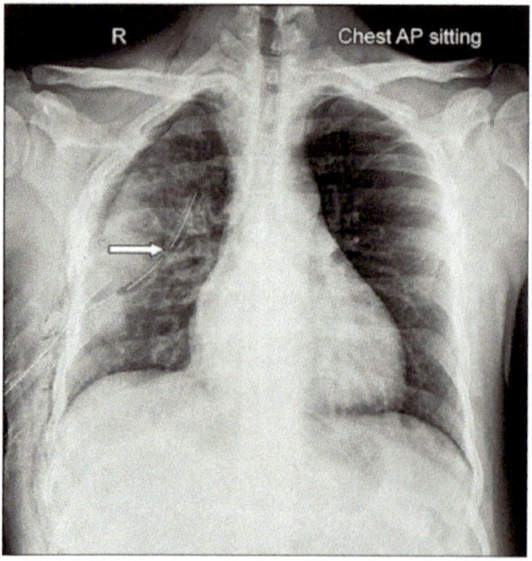

Fig. 3.69: CXR AP view showing right thoracostomy tube.

NASOGASTRIC TUBE (FIG. 3.70)

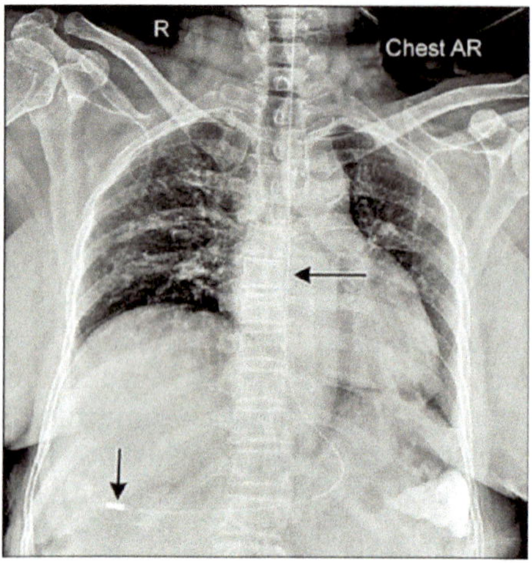

Fig. 3.70: Nasogastric tube should ideally be in distal duodenum.

MULTIPLE CHOICE QUESTIONS

1. **What radiographic feature helps differentiate metastatic nodules from granulomatous nodules?**
   a Spiculated margins
   b. Ground-glass appearance
   c. Central Cavitation
   d. Calcification

2. **Which imaging modality is often used to further evaluate nodular lung disease when chest X-ray findings are inconclusive?**
   a. CT scan
   b. MRI
   c. PET scan
   d. Ultrasound

3. **Which mediastinal mass is typically located anterior to the trachea and heart?**
   a. Thymoma
   b. Neurogenic tumor
   c. Teratoma
   d. Thyroid goiter

4. **What radiographic sign may indicate the presence of an anterior mediastinal mass on chest X-ray?**
   a. Widening of the superior mediastinum
   b. Loss of silhouette sign with the right heart border
   c. Deviation of the trachea to the left
   d. large well-marginated opacity through which the hilum is well seen

5. **Which radiographic finding is characteristic of a lung abscess on chest X-ray?**
   a. Reticular pattern
   b. Air-fluid level within a cavitary lesion
   c. Ground-glass opacities
   d. Pleural effusion

6. What is the typical appearance of a lung abscess on chest X-ray?

a. Reticular pattern
b. Consolidation
c. Nodular opacities
d. Cavitary lesion with surrounding infiltrates

7. Which of the following conditions is often associated with a reticular pattern on chest X-ray?

a. Lung abscess
b. Pulmonary embolism
c. Pulmonary fibrosis
d. Pneumothorax

8. What does a reticular pattern on chest X-ray represent?

a. Atelectasis
b. Infiltrates
c. Scarring or fibrosis
d. Pneumonia

9. Which imaging modality is typically used to confirm the diagnosis of a lung abscess and evaluate its extent?

a. Chest X-ray
b. CT scan
c. MRI
d. Ultrasound

10. What is a solitary pulmonary nodule (SPN)?

a. A single, discrete lesion in the lung parenchyma
b. Multiple lesions scattered throughout the lung fields
c. A large mass involving multiple lobes of the lung
d. A lesion located in the mediastinum

11. Which of the following features suggests a benign etiology for a solitary pulmonary nodule on chest X-ray?

a. Smooth and well-defined margins
b. Irregular and spiculated margins
c. Size greater than 3 cm
d. Central cavitation

12. What is the most common cause of multiple pulmonary nodules on chest X-ray?
   a. Lung cancer
   b. Tuberculosis
   c. Metastatic disease
   d. Pulmonary embolism

13. Which imaging modality is often used to characterize solitary pulmonary nodules and evaluate for malignancy?
   a. Chest X-ray
   b. CT scan
   c. MRI
   d. PET scan

14. What radiographic feature helps differentiate metastatic nodules from granulomatous nodules?
   a. Spiculated margins
   b. Ground-glass appearance
   c. Central cavitation
   d. Calcifications

15. What is the typical appearance of diffuse interstitial disease on chest X-ray?
   a. Hilar enlargement
   b. Reticular or reticulonodular opacities
   c. Consolidation
   d. Solitary pulmonary nodule

16. What is a cavitatory lesion on chest X-ray?
   a. A mass with irregular margins
   b. A round or oval lucency within the lung parenchyma
   c. A fluid-filled structure with an air-fluid level
   d. A thickened bronchial wall

17. Which of the following conditions is commonly associated with cavitatory lesions on chest X-ray?
   a. Tuberculosis
   b. Pulmonary edema
   c. Pleural effusion
   d. Pulmonary fibrosis

18. Which of the following lines/tubes typically appears as a thin, radiopaque line on chest X-ray, positioned along the trachea?
   a. Endotracheal tube
   b. Central venous catheter
   c. Nasogastric tube
   d. Chest tube

19. Which of the following tubes is typically positioned within the esophagus and appears on chest X-ray?
   a. Endotracheal tube
   b. Central venous catheter
   c. Nasogastric tube
   d. Chest tube

20. What is the purpose of a chest tube as seen on chest X-ray?
   a. Administration of medication directly into the lung parenchyma
   b. Monitoring of central venous pressure
   c. Drainage of pleural effusion or pneumothorax
   d. Decompression of tension pneumothorax

21. Which of the following conditions might require the placement of a nasogastric tube?
   a. Respiratory distress syndrome
   b. Gastrointestinal bleeding
   c. Cardiac tamponade
   d. Pulmonary embolism

ANSWERS

1. a	2. a	3. a	4. d
5. b	6. d	7. c	8. c
9. b	10. a	11. a	12. c
13. b	14. d	15. b	16. b
17. a	18. a	19. c	20. c
21. b			

CHAPTER 4

Differential Diagnosis

NORMAL CHEST X-RAY—LANDMARKS

- Cardiac diameter < ½ thoracic width—measured inside ribs
  - Posterior-anterior (PA), inspiratory, erect film
- 1.5 cm change in diameter between inspiration/expiration
- Right heart border
  - Superior vena cava ± azygos vein
  - Right pulmonary artery
  - Right atrium ± left atrium
- Left heart border
  - Aortic arch
  - PA/aortic angle
  - Left PA
  - LA appendage
  - Left ventricle.

"Apparently" Normal CXR

- Breast shadows
- Superior mediastinal masses
- Posterior mediastinal masses—look behind the heart
- Ribs—notching, tumors, cervical ribs
- Bones—clavicles and hyperparathyroidism—Spine
- Labels—dextrocardia
- Beneath diaphragm—gas

- Lungs—small pneumothorax
  - Apical lung disease.

Respiratory Distress and "Normal" CXR

- Pulmonary embolism
- Asthma
- Airway obstruction—Foreign body (FB), secretions, endotracheal tube (ETT) cuff, epiglottis, croup, etc.
- Viral pneumonia.

COIN LESION ON CXR

Single—Common

- 1° carcinoma
- Metastasis
- Hamartoma
- Granuloma
- Tuberculosis (TB).

Multiple—Common

- Metastases
- Granulomata
- Abscesses
- Septic emboli
- Multiple pulmonary emboli
- Hydatid.

Single—Uncommon

- Hydatid
- AV malformation
- Abscess
- Pulmonary embolus/infarction
- Adenoma
- Hematoma
- Bronchogenic cyst

- Wegener's granulomata
- Progressive massive thrombosis.

Multiple—Uncommon
- Arteriovenous (AV) malformation
- Lymphoma
- Wegener's granulomatosis
- Rheumatoid lung.

Features suggestive of *malignancy*
- Male > female
- Smoker
- Age > 70 years ~ 50%
  50–70 years ~ 25%
  < 35 years < 1%
- Increase size < 2 years
- Absence of calcification
- Absence of air bronchogram.

Lobar Consolidation

CXR Appearances

- Homogeneous opacity
- ***No*** "air" bronchogram
- Structural displacement
  - Fissures
  - Vessels
  - Mediastinum, trachea
- Elevation of hemidiaphragm
- Compensatory expansion.

Lobar Pneumonia

- Homogeneous opacity
- "Air" bronchogram
- No structural displacement
  Klebsiella → bulging fissures **(Fig. 4.1)**

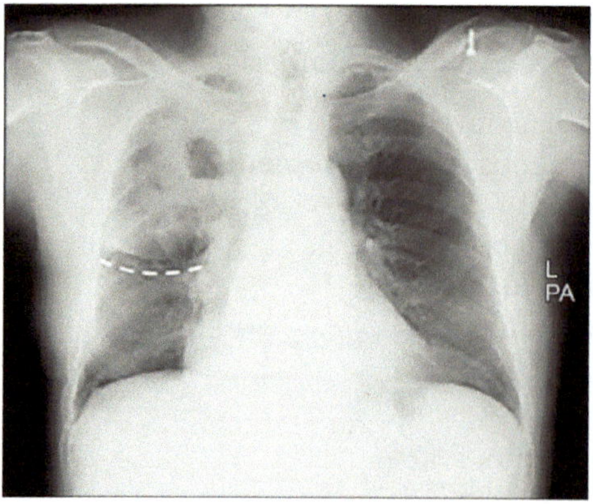

Fig. 4.1: 'Bulging fissure' sign.

- "Paralysis" of hemidiaphragm
- ± pleural effusion, cavitation.

Common Causes

- Sputum retention
- Malposition of ETT
- Mechanical ventilation
- Postoperative
  - Coronary artery bypass grafting (CABG)
  - Upper gastrointestinal tract (GIT)
- Carcinoma, adenoma
- Foreign body.

Bronchopneumonia

- Patchy basal opacities
- "Air" bronchogram
- Clinical signs over affected area.

Butterfly Appearance (Fig. 4.2)

- Pulmonary edema
  - Cardiogenic
  - Noncardiogenic

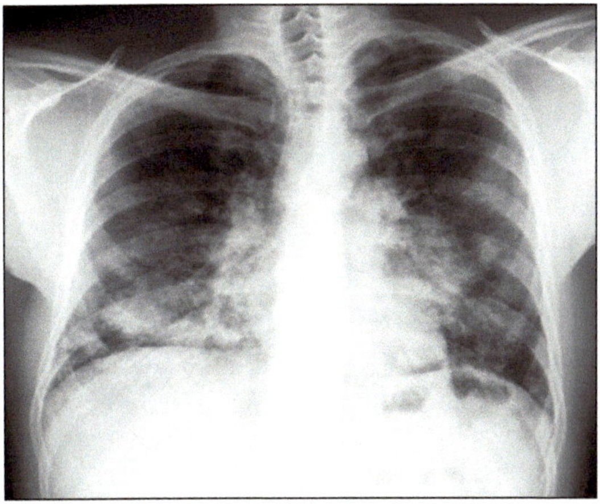

Fig. 4.2: Butterfly appearance.

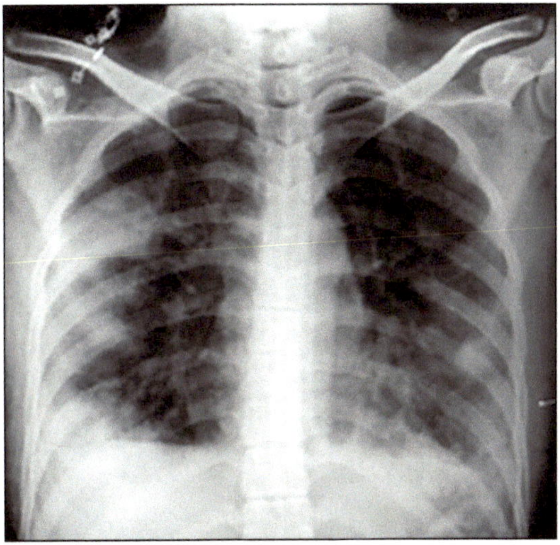

Fig. 4.3: Reverse butterfly appearance.

- Pneumonia
- Alveolar proteinosis
- Lymphoma.

Reversed Butterfly Appearance (Fig. 4.3)

- Pulmonary eosinophilia
- Sarcoidosis.

Bilateral Hilar Enlargement (Fig. 4.4)

- ***Lymphadenopathy***
  - Lymphatic leukemia
  - Lymphoma
  - Hodgkin's disease
  - Carcinoma
    - Renal cell
    - Melanoma
    - Head/neck carcinoma

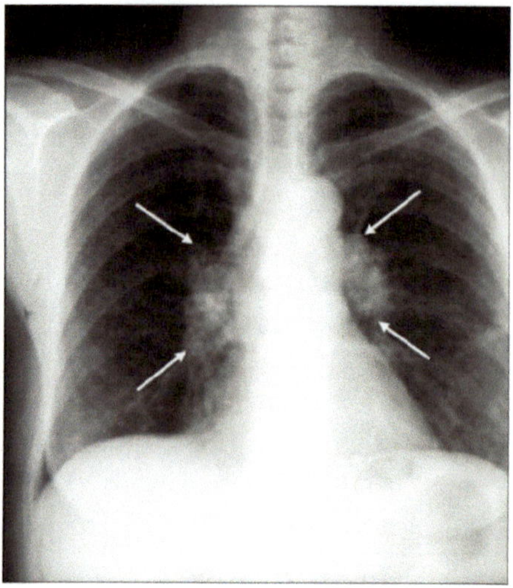

Fig. 4.4: Bilateral hilar lymphadenopathy.

- Sarcoidosis
- Infectious mononucleosis
- Whooping cough
- Primary tuberculosis—rarely, usually unilateral.

- ***Vascular***
  - Pulmonary hypertension—chronic lung disease
    - Multiple pulmonary emboli
    - Primary pulmonary hypertension
  - L → R shunts—atrial septal defect (ASD), ventricular septal defect (VSD)
  - Pulmonary artery dilatation
    - Post-pulmonary stenosis
    - Congenital large pulmonary artery
    - Aneurysm.

Cavitating Lesion on CXR (Fig. 4.5)

- Common
  - Carcinoma
  - Infection—TB, abscess, hydatid
  - Pulmonary emboli, infarct
  - Septic emboli, infarct
- Uncommon
  - Lymphoma
  - Hematoma
  - Bulla
  - Pneumatocele
  - Wegener's
  - Bronchogenic cyst.

Lung Infections

- Lobar/segmental—bacterial, atypical
- Expanding lobar—*Staphylococcus,* gram-negatives, *Klebsiella,* anaerobes
- Cavitating—*Staphylococcus,* gram-negatives, *Klebsiella,* anaerobes, fungi

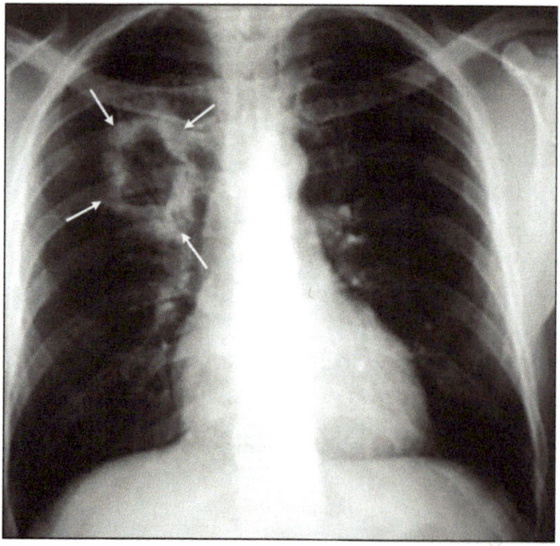

Fig. 4.5: This patient has a large thick-walled cavitating mass in the right lung.

- Generalized alveolar—bacterial, pneumocystis
- Generalized interstitial—viral, TB, atypical, fungal, pneumocystis
- Crescentic—hydatid, fungal
- Effusion—bacterial, TB
- Extrapulmonary—actinomycosis, hydatid
- Pneumothorax—*Staphylococcus, Klebsiella*
- Lymphadenopathy—viral, TB, fungal, actinomycosis.

Apical Disease on CXR

- TB
- Other infections
- Bronchogenic carcinoma—Pancoast's tumor
- Metastases
- Pleural thickening
- Extrapleural disease.

Peribronchial Thickening

- Chronic bronchitis
- Asthma
- Edema
- Bronchiectasis
- Cystic fibrosis.

Diffuse Pulmonary Infiltrates

Note: Divide into ***acute*** or ***chronic***.

1. **Acute**
   - Cardiogenic edema—Left ventricular failure (LVF), mitral stenosis (MS)
   - Acute respiratory distress syndrome (ARDS)—sepsis, trauma, transfusion reaction, fat emboli, etc.
   - Infection—bacterial, viral, fungal, protozoal
   - Hemorrhage—contusions, trauma
     - Infarction, Goodpasture's syndrome, coagulopathy
     - Idiopathic hemosiderosis
   - Aspiration
   - Pulmonary eosinophilia

   Note: In severe chronic obstructive airway disease (COAD) the distribution of edema is patchy.
2. **Subacute**
   - Alveolar proteinosis
   - Lymphangitis carcinomatosis
   - Malignancy—lymphoma, alveolar cell carcinoma
   - Sarcoidosis.
3. **Chronic (upper zones)**
   - Aspergillosis
   - Ankylosing spondylitis, ulcerative colitis
   - Extrinsic fibrosing alveolitis—organic dust inhalation
   - Silicosis
   - Sarcoidosis
   - Tuberculosis
   - Rare—radiotherapy, histiocytosis X.

4. **Chronic (lower zones)**
    - Asbestosis
    - Aspiration—chronic, recurrent
    - Intrinsic fibrosing alveolitis—rheumatoid arthritis (RA), systemic lupus erythematosus (SLE), scleroderma, drugs, etc.
    - Bronchiectasis
    - Chronic bronchitis, COAD
    - Pulmonary eosinophilia—protozoal, drugs
    - Rare-von Recklinghausen's
    - Drugs—amiodarone, bleomycin, busulphan, methysergide, hydralazine, procainamide, sulfonamides.

Upper Lobe

- S—silicosis (progressive massive fibrosis), sarcoidosis
- C—coal workers pneumoconiosis
- H—histiocytosis X
- A—ankylosing spondylitis, aspergillosis
- R—radiation
- T—TB.

Lower Lobe

- R—rheumatoid arthritis
- A—asbestosis
- S-scleroderma
- I—idiopathic
- O—other (busulphan, bleomycin, amiodarone, methotrexate).

Diffuse Interstitial Disease + Mediastinal Lymphadenopathy

- Carcinoma
- Lymphoma
- Sarcoidosis

- Silicosis
- Viral infection.

Diffuse Interstitial Disease + Skeletal Abnormality

- Ribs—scleroderma
- Spine—ankylosing spondylitis
- Shoulder joints—RA, scleroderma, sarcoidosis
    - Hypertrophic pulmonary osteoarthropathy
- Skull—tuberous sclerosis, histiocytosis X.

Miliary Opacities

- Miliary pattern **(Fig. 4.6)**
    - Sarcoidosis
    - Metastases—thyroid, renal, trophoblastic
    - TB
    - Silicosis
    - Chickenpox
    - Fibrosing alveolitis
    - Pneumoconiosis.

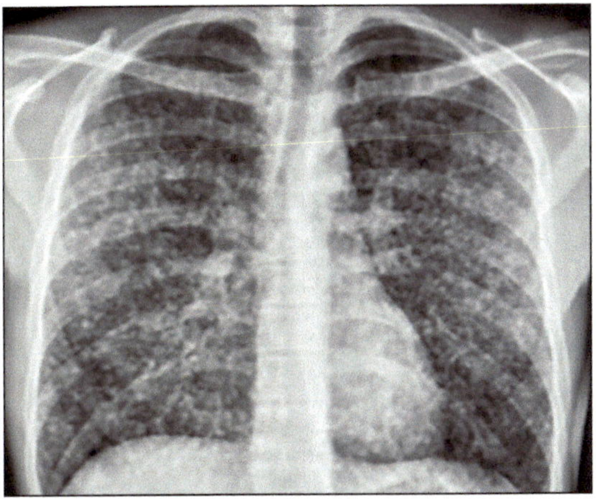

Fig. 4.6: Miliary pattern.

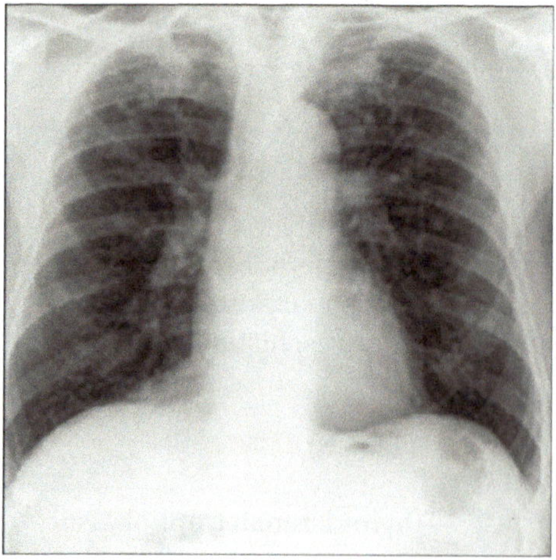

Fig. 4.7: Dense nodules.

- Dense nodules **(Fig. 4.7)**
  - Silicosis
  - Chronic hemosiderosis
  - Metal
  - Microlithiasis.

Cardiophrenic Angle Mass

- Fat pad—obesity, lipoma, steroids
- Hernia of Morgagni
- Pericardial cyst
- Pericardial tumor.

Hyperinflated Lungs

- ***Bilateral hyperinflation***
  - COAD
  - Asthma
  - α_1-antitrypsin deficiency

    - Cystic fibrosis
    - Bronchiolitis
    - Aspergillosis.
- ***Unilateral hyperinflation***
    - Foreign body with hyperinflation
    - Pneumothorax
    - Large pulmonary embolus
    - Lung cyst, bullae
    - Unilateral emphysema
    - Post-lobectomy hyperinflation.
- ***Apparent unilateral hyperinflation***
    - Rotated normal CXR
    - Increased density on other side
    - Absent breast
    - Absent pectoral muscle—congenital, surgical
    - Scoliosis.

Pulmonary Oligemia

- Low cardiac output
- R → L shunt-Fallot's, Ebstein's, trilogy
- Pulmonary artery banding.

Pulmonary Plethora

- Features
    - ≤ 1:1 distribution of vessel diameter—capillary filtration venous hypertension >1
    - Increase number of hilar vessels
- Causes
    - Hyperdynamic circulation
        - Polycythemia
        - Thyrotoxicosis
        - Fluid overload
    - L→ R shunt—ASD, VSD, patent ductus arteriosus (PDA)
        - Partial anomalous pulmonary venous drainage

- Bidirectional shunt
  - Transposition, truncus arteriosus
  - Partial anomalous pulmonary venous drainage.

Large Lesions on CXR

- ***Common***
  - Tumor
  - Infection
  - TB
  - Hydatid
  - Encased effusion
  - Progressive massive fibrosis.
- ***Uncommon***
  - Infection
  - Bronchogenic cyst
  - Pulmonary sequestration—aortic, not pulmonary artery supply.
- ***"Air-crescent" sign → cavity + (Fig. 4.8)***
  - Fungal infection
  - Clot

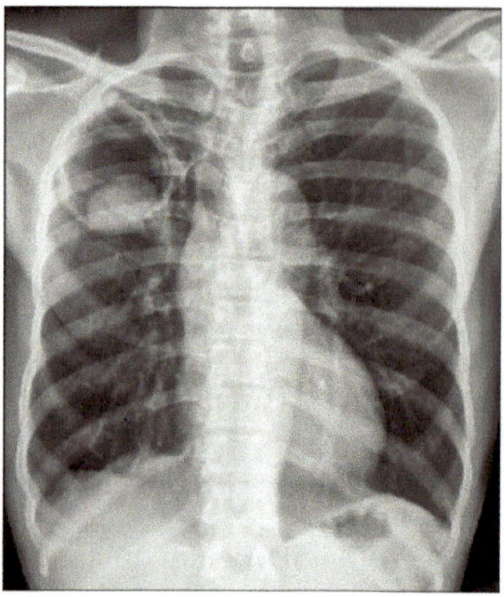

Fig. 4.8: Air-crescent sign.

- Tumor
- Hydatid.

Mediastinal Masses

- ***Commonest***
  - Fat deposition—obesity, lipoma, steroids
  - Vascular
- ***Anterior***
  - Thymus
  - Thyroid
  - Other tumor—teratoma, dermoid cyst, lipoma
  - Ascending aortic aneurysm
  - Lymphadenopathy.
- ***Middle***
  - Heart
  - Aortic arch aneurysm
  - Pulmonary vessels
  - Trachea
  - Bronchogenic cyst
  - Lymphadenopathy.
- ***Posterior***
  - Descending aortic aneurysm
  - Hiatus hernia
  - Diaphragmatic hernia
  - Lymphadenopathy
  - Neuroma
  - Neuroblastoma
  - Enterogenic cyst.

Calcification on CXR

- ***Localized calcification***
  - Tuberculosis
  - Hematoma
  - Hamartoma—popcorn calcification

  - Teratoma
  - Rarely—sarcoid, asbestosis.
- ***Diffuse calcification***
  - Post-varicella pneumonia
  - Tuberculosis
  - Histoplasmosis
  - Silicosis
  - Chronic hemosiderosis.
- ***Hilar calcification***
  - Lymph nodes
    - Tuberculosis
    - Silicosis
    - Sarcoidosis
    - Histoplasmosis
  - Pulmonary atherosclerosis.
- ***"Eggshell" calcification***
  - Silicosis
  - Sarcoid
  - Scleroderma
  - Anthracosis
  - Lymphoma after radiotherapy
  - Amyloid
  - Histoplasmosis.
- ***Pleural calcification***
  - Tuberculosis
  - Empyema
  - Hemothorax
  - Asbestosis.

Extrapleural Mass on CXR

- Osteomyelitis
- Actinomycosis
- Hydatid
- Tumor 1° or 2°
- Myeloma

- Fracture
- Extramedullary hematopoiesis.

Pleural Effusion

Note: > 300 mL

- Loss of costophrenic angle
- Upper border meniscus
- Homogeneous opacity obscures heart border and diaphragm
- Mediastinal shift
- Increase distance between lung and stomach gas on left
- ***Lateral decubitus*** reveals change in meniscus and useful for small or unusual effusion.

Massive Pleural Effusion

- Post-thoracotomy/pneumonectomy
- Tumor
- Empyema
- TB
- Hemothorax
- Ruptured esophagus.

Rib Notching

- Coarctation of aorta
- Inferior vena cava (IVC) obstruction
- Neurofibromas
- Tuberous sclerosis
- Idiopathic.

CXR: Specific Pictures

Aspiration Pneumonitis (Fig. 4.9)

- Normal CXR—small aspiration or too early
- Linear (interstitial) densities

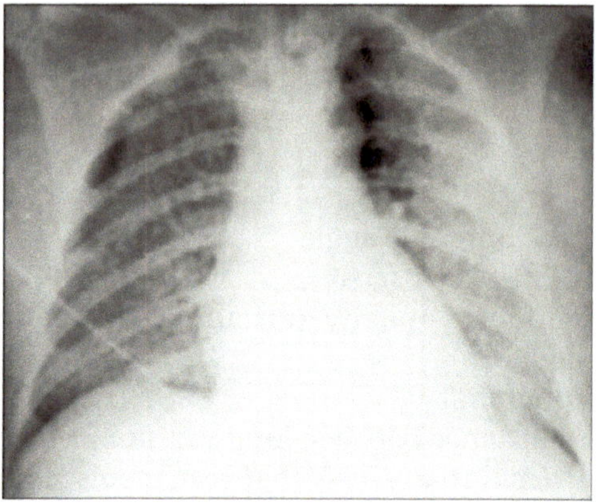

Fig. 4.9: Chest X ray showing aspiration pneumonitis.

- Nodular (alveolar) or patchy infiltrates
- Lobar consolidation/collapse
- Noncardiogenic pulmonary edema (ARDS).

Chronic Obstructive Pulmonary Disease (Fig. 4.10)

- PA or AP
  - Flattening of diaphragm
  - Thin heart shadow
  - Attenuation of vessels
  - Vessels "pulled" down → "like drooping moustache"
  - Bullae
  - Bulging of lung edges → between ribs and around heart.
- Lateral
  - Flattening of diaphragm
  - ↑ AP diameter
  - ↑ retrosternal air shadow
  - Bullae.
- Etiology
  - Smoking
  - Chronic asthma

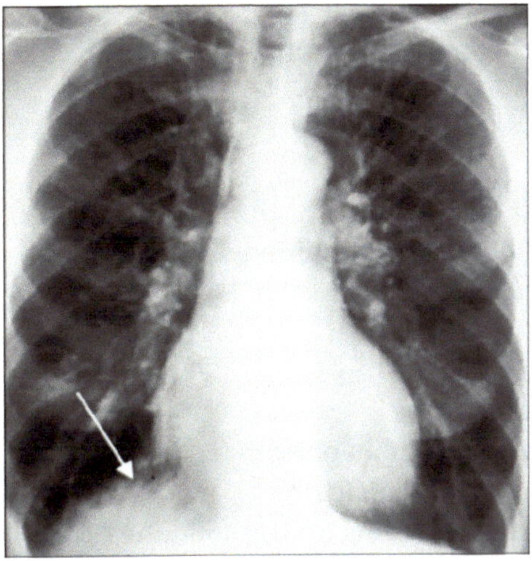

Fig. 4.10: Chest X-ray of a patient showing COPD.

- α_1-antitrypsin deficiency
- Chronic dust/pollution exposure
- Cystic fibrosis.

Sarcoidosis

- Bilateral hilar lymphadenopathy
- Opacities spreading from hilum into parenchyma
- Miliary opacities—sarcoid nodules
- Paratracheal lymphadenopathy.

Tuberculosis

- Unilateral hilar lymphadenopathy—1°TB ± calcification
- Primary lesion in middle lobe or apex of lower lobe
- Subapical lesion—
  - Opacity
  - Cavity
  - ± calcification

- Bronchopneumonic changes
- Miliary opacities—obscure normal lung markings
- Acute lung injury, ARDS.

Carcinoma

- ***Possible CXR features***
  - Consolidation/"pneumonia"
  - Apical mass ± rib erosion
  - Cavitating lesion
  - Lung abscess
  - Lobar collapse
  - Paralyzed hemidiaphragm
  - Hilar lymphadenopathy
  - Miliary shadowing from secondaries.
- ***Lung metastases***
  - Canon-ball opacities **(Fig. 4.12)**
  - Miliary opacities **(Figs. 4.11A and B)**
  - Numerous ill-defined opacities
  - Kerley B lines—obstructed lymphatics, no cardiomegaly.

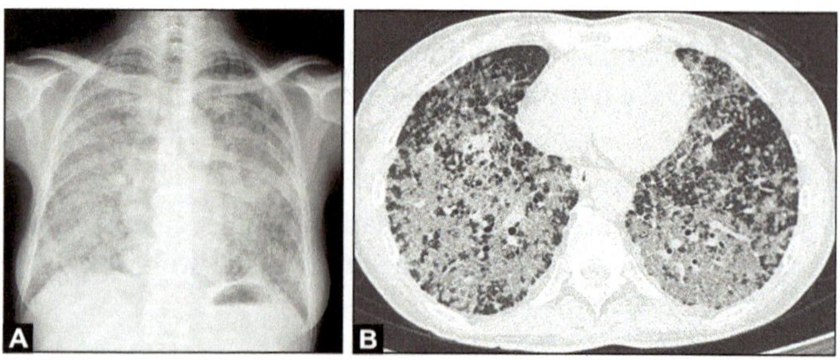

Figs. 4.11A and B: (A) Chest Xray showing miliary opacities; (B) Corresponding CT image showing miliary opacities.

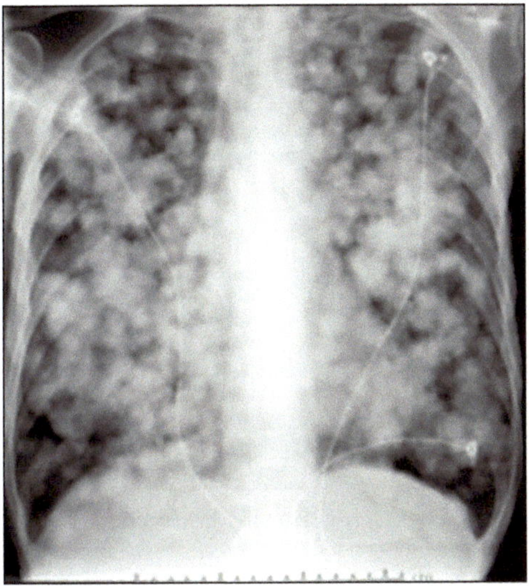

Fig. 4.12: Chest X ray showing canon ball opacities.

- ***Central mass*** →
  - Squamous ~ 40%
  - Anaplastic ~ 40% → large or small cell.
- ***Peripheral mass***
  - Alveolar cell
  - Adenocarcinoma
  - Pancoast's.

Pulmonary Embolus (Fig. 4.13)

- Normal CXR
- Transient unilateral increase in lung lucency
  - Westermark's sign—due to generalized vasoconstriction
- Unilateral peripheral translucent area
- Pleurally-based, wedge-shaped or 'D'-shaped opacity on lateral CXR

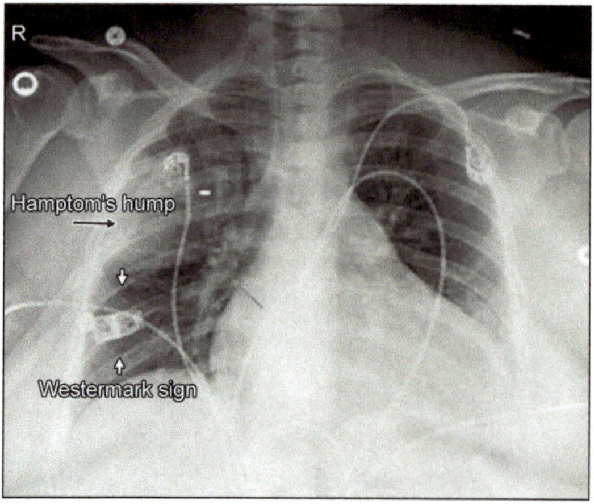

Fig. 4.13: Chest X ray showing pulmonary embolism.

  - Hampton's hump
  - Hazy opacity on PA CXR
- Pleural effusion
- Linear atelectasis
- Raised hemidiaphragm
- Enlargement of hilum
- RV enlargement, azygos vein dilatation
- Rarely calcification.

Pulmonary Arterial Hypertension

- Features
  - Enlarged, well-defined hilar vessels—arise from hilum
  - ± calcification
  - Rapid tapering of vessels
  - Very few peripheral vascular markings
  - No effusions or Kerley lines, i.e., no signs of LVF
  - Cardiomegaly—RV and RA
  - Prominent IVC and SVC
  - CXR changes are *late*.

- Causes
  - L → R shunt
  - Pulmonary embolism
  - Cor pulmonale
  - Mitral stenosis
  - Idiopathic pulmonary arterial hypertension (PAH).

Pulmonary Venous Hypertension

- Features = upper lobe venous diversion
  - UL > LL veins
  - First interspace vessel > 3 mm
  - Any segmental artery > 5 mm

Note: ↑ magnification on portable AP films, may exceed these limits.

- Causes
  - LVF
  - Mitral stenosis
  - Left atrial—myxoma, tumor, thrombus
  - Cor triatriatum
  - Anomalous pulmonary venous drainage
  - Constrictive pericarditis
  - Pulmonary venous fibrosis or thrombosis.

Fat Embolus

- Normal CXR in 88%
- Patchy consolidation
- Right heart failure
- Bilateral diffuse infiltrates—ARDS

Lung Infiltrates in Renal Failure

- Septicemia
- Bacterial pneumonia
- Cardiogenic shock
- Acute lung injury

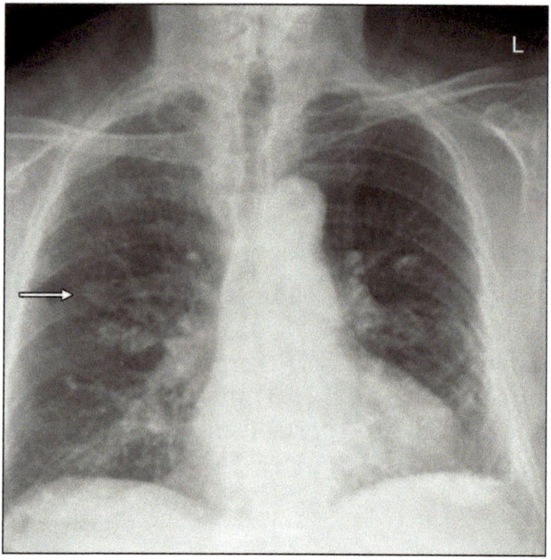

Fig. 4.14: Chest X ray showing plaques in a patient with asbestosis.

  - ARDS
  - Multiple organ system failure (MOSF)
- Atypical pneumonia—*Legionella*
- Autoimmune disease
  - Goodpasture's syndrome
  - Polyarteritis
  - SLE
  - Wegener's granulomatosis
- Drug effects.

Mesothelioma/Asbestosis (Fig. 4.14 and Table 4.1)

- Exposure to asbestos fibers
- Restrictive lung deficit
- Radiological changes.

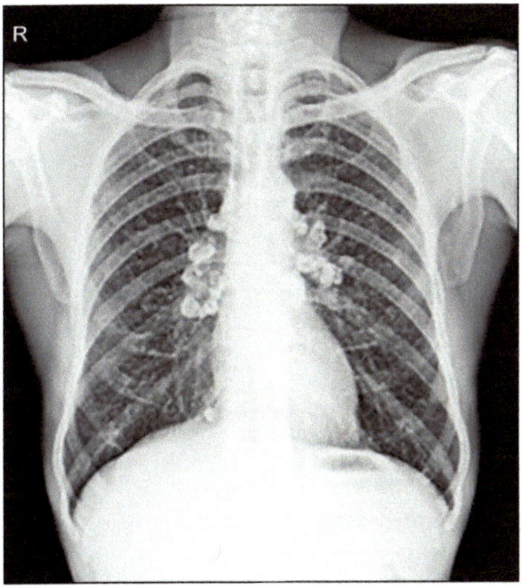

Fig. 4.15: Chest X ray-egg shell calcifications.

CXR patterns of presentation
- Peripheral opacities
- Geographical plaques and calcification
- Pulmonary fibrosis
- Bronchogenic carcinoma.

Silicosis (Table 4.1)

- Numerous small nodules—upper zones
- Pulmonary fibrosis—upper zones
- Egg-shell calcification—DDX sarcoid **(Fig. 4.15)**.

TABLE 4.1: Differences between asbestosis and silicosis.

Asbestosis	*Silicosis*
Lower lobe fibrosis	Upper lobe fibrotic changes
Progressive massive fibrosis—uncommon	Progressive massive fibrosis—common

Asbestosis	*Silicosis*
Mesothelioma	Bronchogenic carcinoma
Pleural calcifications	Calcific hilar nodes
Tuberculosis—uncommon	Tuberculosis—common

CXR: CARDIAC

Heart Size

- ***Small heart***
  - Hyperinflated lungs—asthma, emphysema
  - Hypovolemia
  - Addison's disease
  - Cachexia, anorexia
  - Normal variant
- ***Massive enlargement***
  - Mitral valve disease
  - Pericardial effusion
  - Cardiomyopathy
  - Ebstein's anomaly
- ***Moderate enlargement*** → above plus
  - Ischemic heart disease
  - Hypertensive heart disease
  - Valvular heart disease
  - Cardiomyopathy
  - Pericardial tumor, cyst
  - Factitious
    - Supine or AP film
    - Raised hemidiaphragms
- ***LA enlargement***
  - Mitral valve disease
  - LVF
  - VSD
  - PDA

  (LVF, VSD, PDA) → pulmonary blood flow and LA volume overload

Congestive Cardiac Failure (CCF)

- Cardiomegaly
- Pulmonary congestion → UL ≥ LL vessels
- Prominent lymphatics
  - Blurring of hilar vessels—dilated lymphatics
  - Visible lymphatics—Kerley A and B lines
- Interstitial edema → reticular pattern, Kerley C lines
- Alveolar edema
  - Diffuse patchy opacities
  - "Cotton-wool" opacities around bronchi → LL > ML > UL
  - Blurring of cardiac borders
- Pleural effusion, fluid in lobar fissures

Lung fields reflect cardiac function better than heart size does.

Pulmonary Edema

- ***Chronic/cardiogenic***
  - Septal lines—Kerley's lines
  - Diffuse reticular pattern
  - Perivascular and peribronchial cuffing
  - Subpleural thickening and edema
  - Perihilar and basal infiltrates
  - Upper lobe venous distension
  - Pleural effusion
  - Air bronchogram rare.
- ***Acute and/or noncardiogenic,*** e.g., ARDS
  - Patchy alveolar edema—not hilar
  - Air bronchograms
  - With well-defined cardiac borders and
  - No lymphatics nor venous congestion visible
  - Normal cardiac and PA size

Kerley's lines: A and B → septal lymphatics

A. Large, 4–6 cm, irregular, radiate from hilum to upper lobes
B. Short 1–2 cm, horizontal, basal, touch pleural margin
   Transient—fluid
   Permanent—MS, tumor, lymphangitis, pneumoconiosis
C. Fine curvilinear, often generalized, giving reticular pattern.

Pulmonary Edema: Acute

Note: Signs usually present in acute pulmonary edema, alveolar and interstitial edema with:

- Normal heart size
- Normal PA size
- No venous congestion
- Normal size azygos vein
- Absence of Kerley's lines.

Pulmonary Edema: Unilateral

- Pulmonary embolus—on unaffected side
- Re-expansion of collapsed lung or pneumothorax
- Unilateral lung cysts or emphysema—on unaffected side
- Severe cardiomegaly and congestive cardiac failure (CCF) → R-sided edema (left PA compressed)
- Patient in lateral position—gravity, dependent side
- Aspiration pneumonitis
- Congenital heart disease and shunt, e.g., Fallot's.

Mitral Stenosis

- Signs of high pulmonary venous pressure
    - Kerly A and B septal lines
    - Prominent minor fissure with fluid
    - Upper lobe venous distension
    - Pulmonary edema
    - Dilated left atrium → see over
    - Straight left heart border and increase in LA appendage

- Other features
  - Calcified mitral valve
  - Dilated pulmonary arteries > aortic diameter
  - ***Normal*** heart size in uncomplicated cases Undersized LV but abnormal function.

Left Atrial Dilatation

- PA or AP CXR
  - Double heart border on right
  - Loss of LA appendage "trough"
  - Splayed carina
  - Cardiomegaly
  - Esophageal displacement—NGT or barium swallow
  - ± pulmonary edema
- Lateral CXR
  - Posterior bulging of the cardiac border.

Fallot's Tetralogy ('Boot' shaped heart) (Fig. 4.16)

- Apex of the heart raised above level of hemidiaphragm
- Pulmonary oligemia
- Small pulmonary arteries
- Dilated aorta.

Atrial Septal Defect (ASD)

- LA dilatation
- RA dilatation
- Large pulmonary artery
- Dilated UL and LL veins
- Small aortic arch < PA diameter

Eisenmenger's Syndrome

Definition: Reversal of right → left shunt as a result of pulmonary hypertension

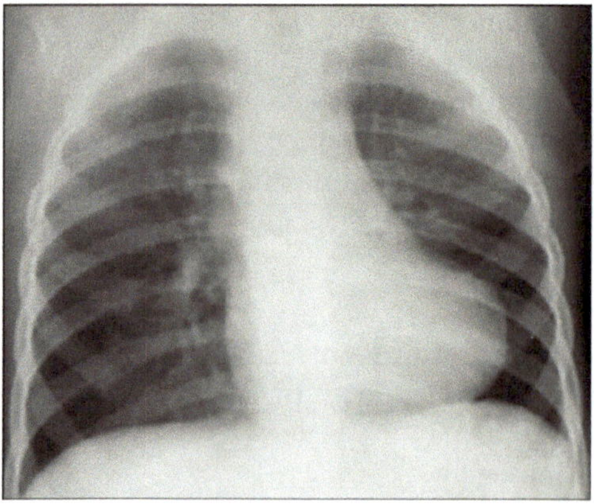

Fig. 4.16: Chest X ray showing boot shaped heart.

1. Large dilated main pulmonary arteries
2. Oligemia of peripheral lung fields
3. Small aortic shadow.

Coarctation of the Aorta

- Rib notching → 3rd–7th ribs
- "Wasting" or "3-sign" on descending aorta—pre/post-stenotic dilatation **(Fig. 4.17)**
  - Prominent left subclavian artery
  - Cardiomegaly → LVH.

Pericardial Effusion

Note: X-ray changes late → > 200 mL required

- "Water-bag" cardiomegaly, large globular cardiac shadow **(Fig. 4.18)**
- Acute angle between cardiac shadow and hemidiaphragms
- Clear heart border—no movement of heart seen to blur film
- Symmetrical cardiac enlargement
- Clear lungs—no left ventricular failure (LVF).

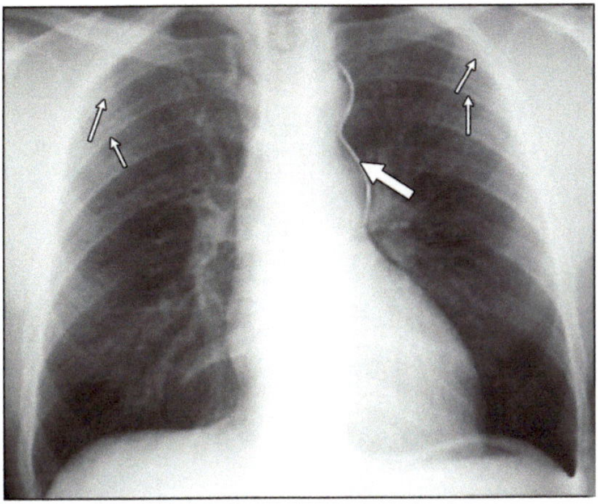

Fig. 4.17: Chest X ray showing '3' sign (Thick arrow).

Constrictive Pericarditis

- Cardiomegaly
- Pericardial calcification—especially oblique and lateral
- More common with:
  - Chronic idiopathic
  - Chronic renal failure
  - Rheumatoid arthritis
  - Neoplastic
  - Tuberculosis
  - Irradiation.

Patent Ductus Arteriosus

1–5 as for ASD

6. L atrial dilatation
7. R atrial dilatation
8. R ventricular dilatation
9. Large pulmonary artery

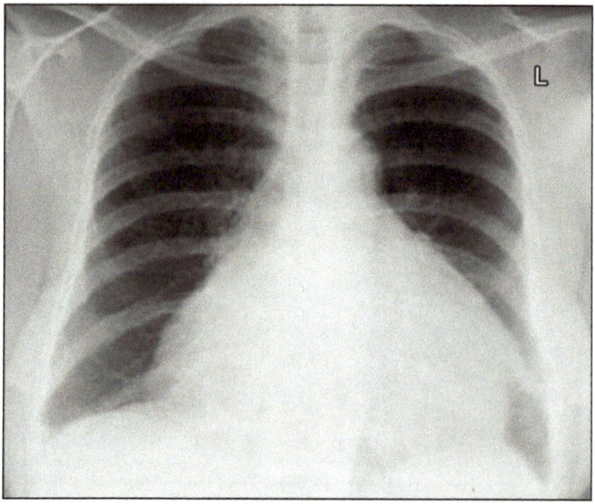

Fig. 4.18: Chest X-ray showing cardiomegaly-'Water Bag' sign.

10. Dilated UL and LL veins
11. Large aorta.

Right Heart Failure

- Cardiomegaly—RV + RA
- SVC and azygos vein distension
- ± Pulmonary artery prominence
- **No** alveolar edema.

MULTIPLE CHOICE QUESTIONS

1. **Which of the following features is not consistent with right heart failure?**
   a. Cardiomegaly
   b. Prominent pulmonary artery
   c. Alveolar edema
   d. SVC and azygous vein distension

2. **Which of the following have "Revere butterfly appearance" on chest X-ray?**
   a. Pulmonary edema
   b. Pulmonary eosinophilia
   c. Lymphoma
   d. Alveolar proteinosis

3. **Which of the following diseases is not consistent with massive enlargement of heart?**
   a. Mitral valve disease
   b. Pericardial effusion
   c. Ebstein's anomaly
   d. Addison's disease

4. **Which of the following features is not consistent with acute pulmonary edema on chest X-ray?**
   a. Kerley's lines
   b. Normal heart size
   c. Normal pulmonary artery size
   d. Patchy alveolar edema

5. **Which of the following can show classical 'air-crescent' sign on chest X-ray, except?**
   a. Fungal infection
   b. Clot
   c. Hydatid
   d. Bronchogenic cyst

6. Which of the following conditions is NOT typically included in the differential diagnosis of posterior mediastinal masses of the lung?
   a. Thymoma
   b. Hiatus hernia
   c. Lymphoma
   d. Neurogenic tumors

ANSWERS

1. c	2. b	3. d	4. a
5. d	6. a		

CHAPTER 5

Chest X-ray Correlations with HRCT

INTRODUCTION

Plain radiography remains the standard for screening and to some extent detection of diffuse pulmonary processes in an ICU setting.

One of the main limitations of plain radiography in the evaluation of diffuse pulmonary parenchymal disease is the superimposition of structures due to the projectional format of that imaging method.

As computed tomography offers an unobstructed cross-sectional view of the thorax, its role has become a main stay in defining early detection and characterization of diffuse parenchymal lung diseases.

After more than a decade of technical developments, thin-section high resolution computed tomography (HRCT) has emerged as an accurate method to assess diffuse abnormalities of the pulmonary parenchyma.

In this chapter, CXR and HRCT findings are correlated to give the reader a comprehensive understanding while they attempt to interpret X-rays in training.

CASE 1

Diagnosis: Solitary pulmonary nodule.

Chest X-ray PA and axial NECT and coronal contrast reformats show the left lung upper lobe nodule with a calcific speck **(Fig. 5.1)**.

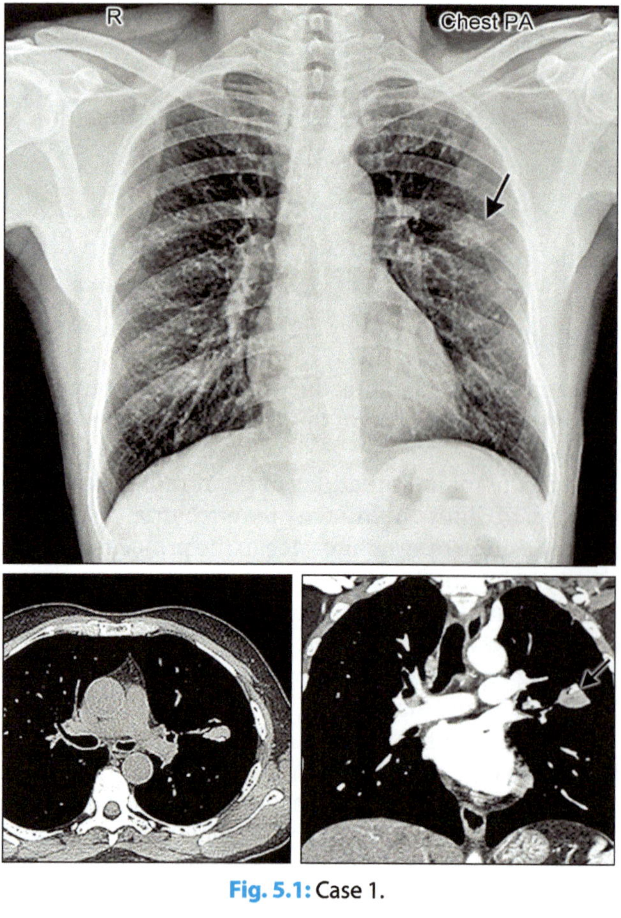

Fig. 5.1: Case 1.

Note: CT helps in assessment of location, enhancement and matrix characteristics.

CASE 2

Diagnosis: Allergic bronchopulmonary aspergillosis (ABPA).

Chest X-ray and HRCT images showing central bronchiectasis with proximal tubular opacities suggestive of ABPA. CT sections show the exact anatomical location and associated parenchymal changes in the form of bronchiolar nodules **(Fig. 5.2)**.

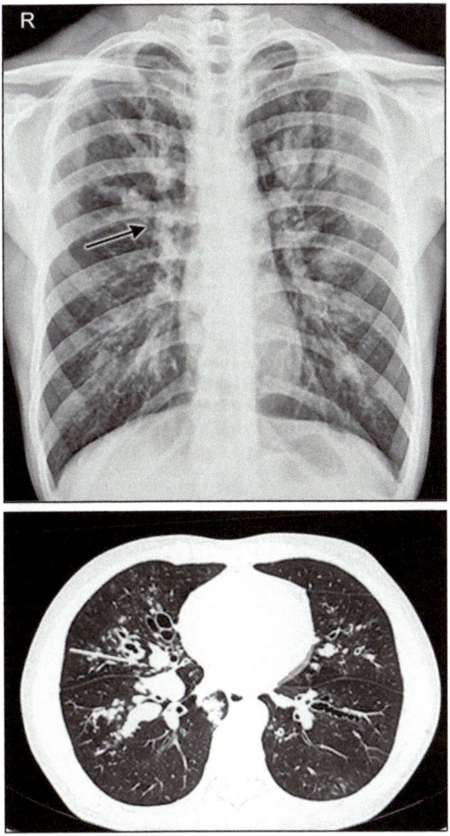

Fig. 5.2: Case 2.

CASE 3

Diagnosis: Provisional diagnosis of pneumocystis pneumonia (pneumocystis pneumonia (PCP).

Chest X-ray showing bilateral hazy opacities with an apparent mid-basal gradient in a febrile immunocompromised patient, HRCT section showing ground-glass opacities **(Fig. 5.3)**.

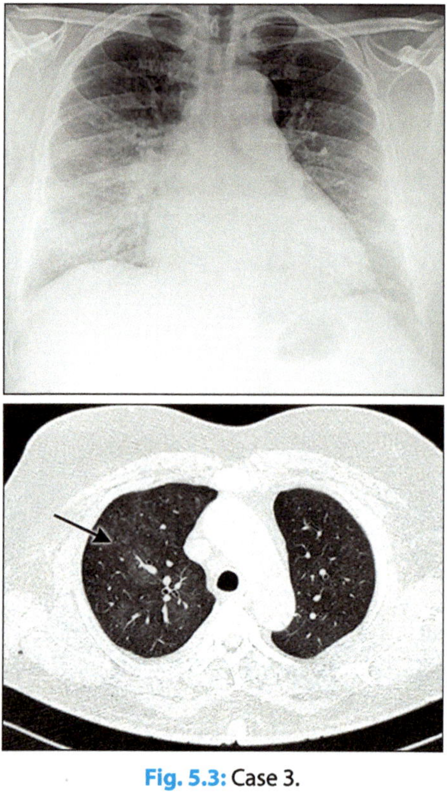

Fig. 5.3: Case 3.

CASE 4

Diagnosis: Situs inversus, CT shows the bronchovascular relations easily, and also helps in ruling out early bronchiectasis as in this patient with Kartagener's syndrome **(Fig. 5.4)**.

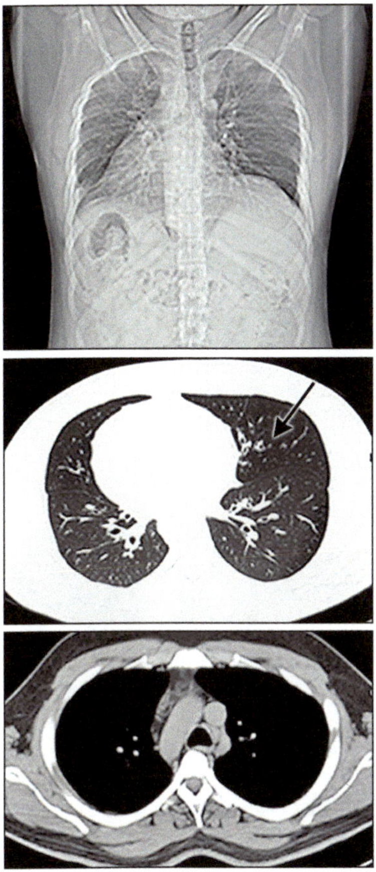

Fig. 5.4: Case 4.

CASE 5

Diagnosis: Consolidation.

Chest X-ray and coronal HRCT reformats in minimum intensity projection showing right upper lobe consolidation. CT reformats helps to trace even the segmental bronchi **(Fig. 5.5)**.

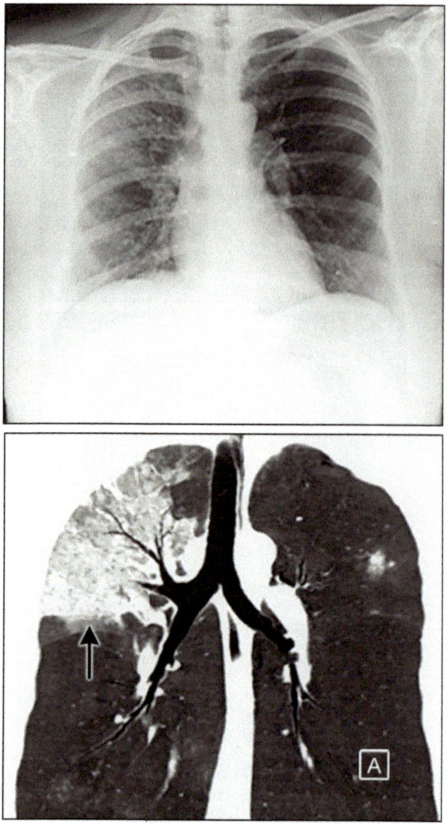

Fig. 5.5: Case 5.

CASE 6

Diagnosis: Benign lesions like bronchogenic/duplication cyst.

Chest X-ray shows a left apical well-marginated smooth opacity, CT images show the matrix of the lesion and its relationship with adjacent structures like esophagus, trachea and neck vessels **(Fig. 5.6)**.

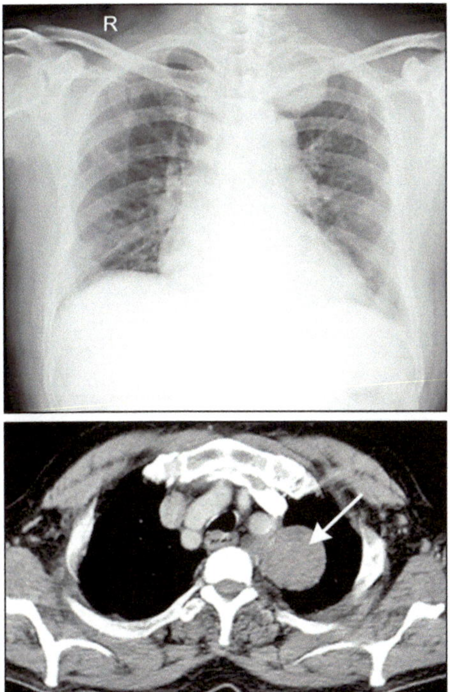

Fig. 5.6: Case 6.

CASE 7

Diagnosis: Interstitial fibrosis—secondary to scleroderma.

Chest X-ray shows bilateral reticular changes and thin-walled lucent opacities in a basal gradient, CT section shows bilateral honeycombing with dilated esophagus which prompted the correct diagnosis **(Fig. 5.7)**.

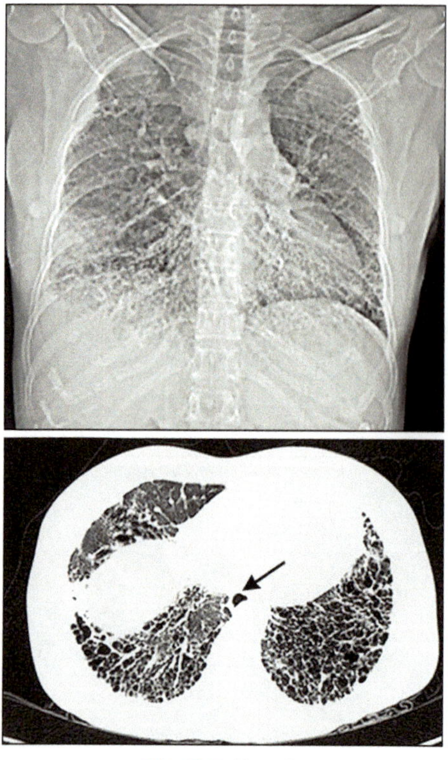

Fig. 5.7: Case 7.

CASE 8

Diagnosis: Possible neurogenic tumor.

Chest X-ray shows right upper zone paratracheal opacity with smooth margin. Axial CECT shows the exact location and matrix of the lesion located in the right costovertebral junction **(Fig. 5.8)**.

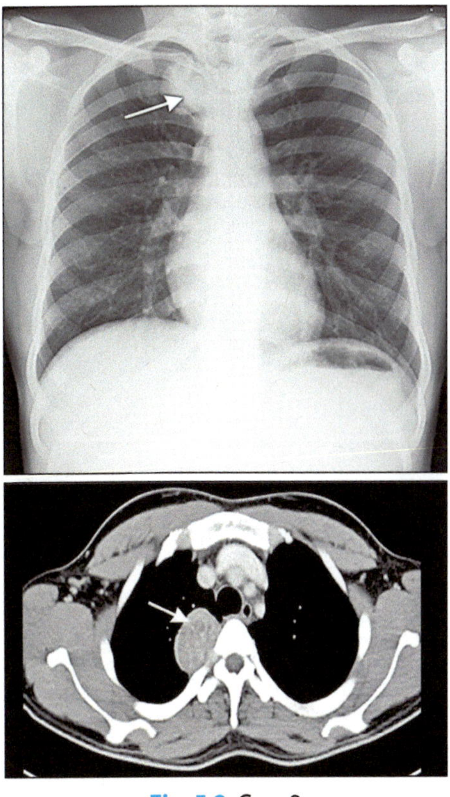

Fig. 5.8: Case 8.

CASE 9

Diagnosis: Suspected chronic eosinophilic pneumonia.

Chest X-ray shows bilateral peripheral consolidative changes, HRCT section shows the distribution of the peripheral subpleural consolidative disease process and matrix change **(Fig. 5.9)**.

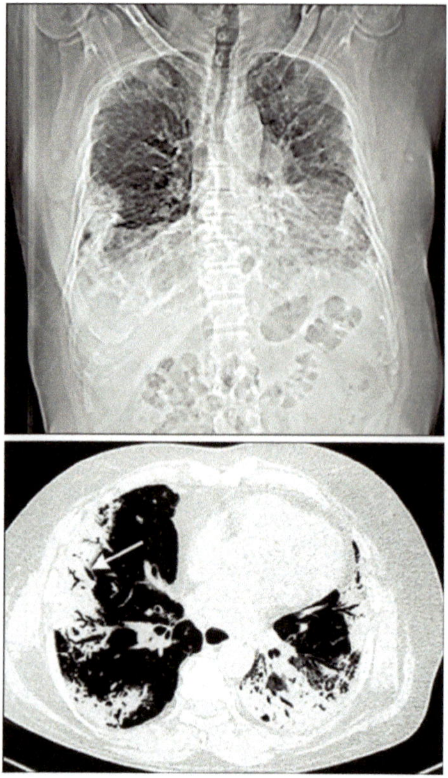

Fig. 5.9: Case 9.

CASE 10

Diagnosis: Subacute extrinsic allergic alveolitis.

Chest X-ray shows minimal doubtful bilateral hazy opacities, HRCT sections show centrilobular nodular opacities which are characteristic finding in extrinsic allergic alveolitis (EAA) **(Fig. 5.10)**.

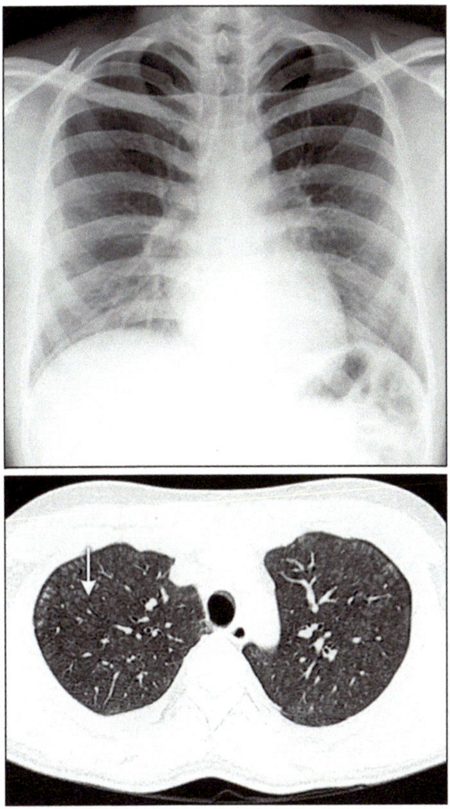

Fig. 5.10: Case 10.

CASE 11

Diagnosis: Active Koch's lesion.

Chest X-ray shows right mid-zone consolidation with cavitary changes, HRCT image shows cavitary consolidation with adjacent transbronchial nodular spread in both lungs **(Fig. 5.11)**.

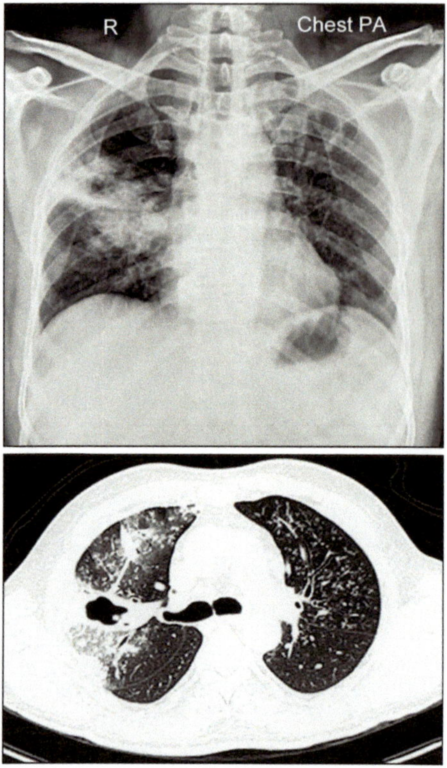

Fig. 5.11: Case 11.

CASE 12

Diagnosis: Pulmonary edema.

Chest X-ray showing bilateral perihilar opacities, HRCT lung showing confluent alveolar opacities. CXR is useful in the critical care setting where repeat images can be obtained to assess dynamic changes **(Fig. 5.12)**.

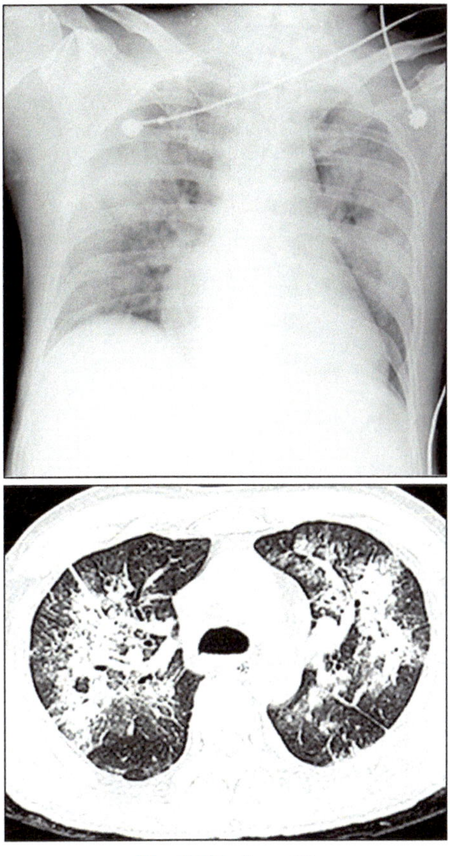

Fig. 5.12: Case 12.

CASE 13

Diagnosis: Postoperative infective consolidation (most lesions resolved on 1 week follow-up).

Chest X-ray and HRCT lungs showing multifocal consolidative changes, HRCT helps in assessing the amount of aerated lung in these cases with extensive opacities and helps in planning invasive treatment if needed **(Fig. 5.13)**.

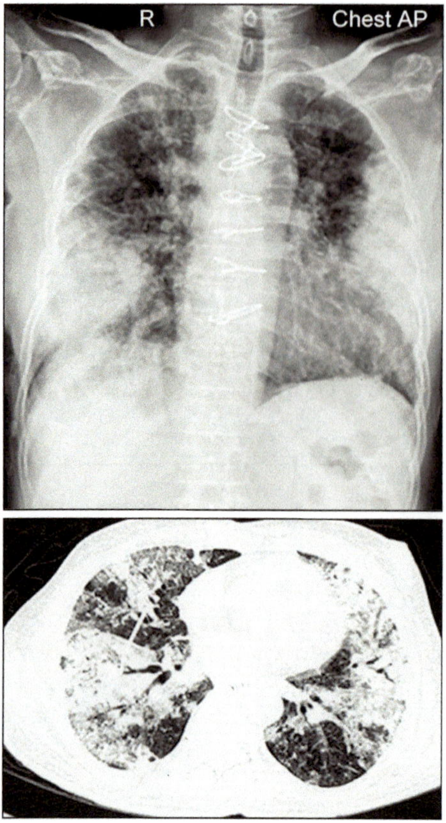

Fig. 5.13: Case 13.

CASE 14

Diagnosis: Pulmonary microlithiasis.

Chest X-ray shows bilateral dense reticulonodular shadows, HRCT lung in bone window setting shows typical dense nodularities **(Fig. 5.14)**.

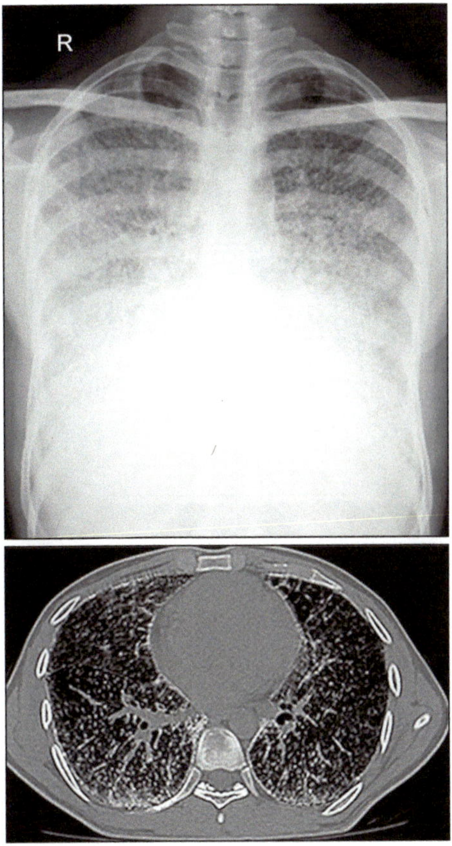

Fig. 5.14: Case 14.

CASE 15

Diagnosis: Miliary Koch's.

Chest X-ray in a febrile patient shows suspicious hard to perceive miliary nodules. HRCT lungs shows discrete diffuse miliary nodules **(Fig. 5.15)**.

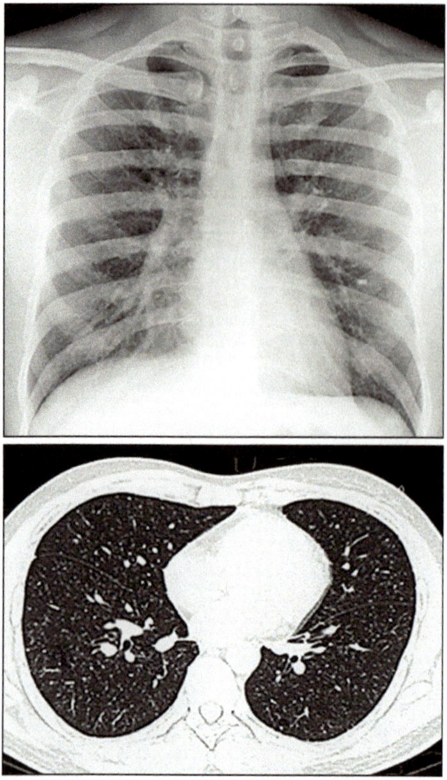

Fig. 5.15: Case 15.

CASE 16

Diagnosis: Infective nodules.

Chest X-ray AP projection in a febrile diabetic patient with respiratory distress showing multiple random nodules. CT lung shows the distribution of these nodules well. In the acute setting based on the distribution of nodules and associated features like cavitation and halo sign it is possible to characterize the nature of infections **(Fig. 5.16)**.

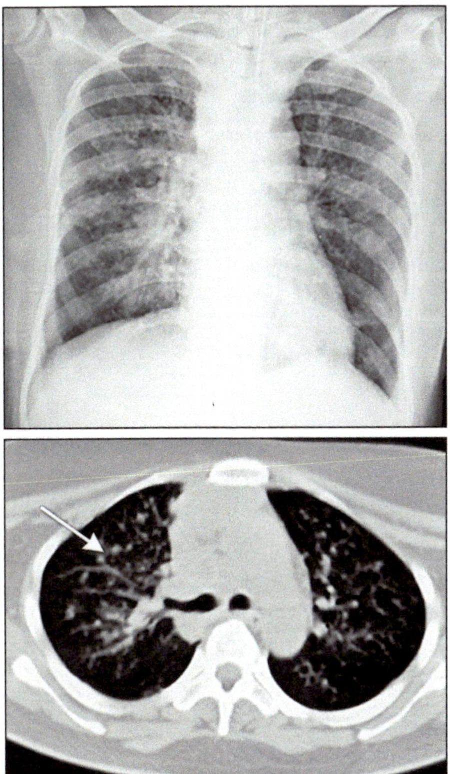

Fig. 5.16: Case 16.

CASE 17

Diagnosis: Koch's lymphadenopathy.

Chest X-ray shows right hilar and paratracheal soft tissue opacities suggestive of nodes.

CECT shows typical hypodense rim enhancing nodes characteristic of Koch's **(Fig. 5.17)**.

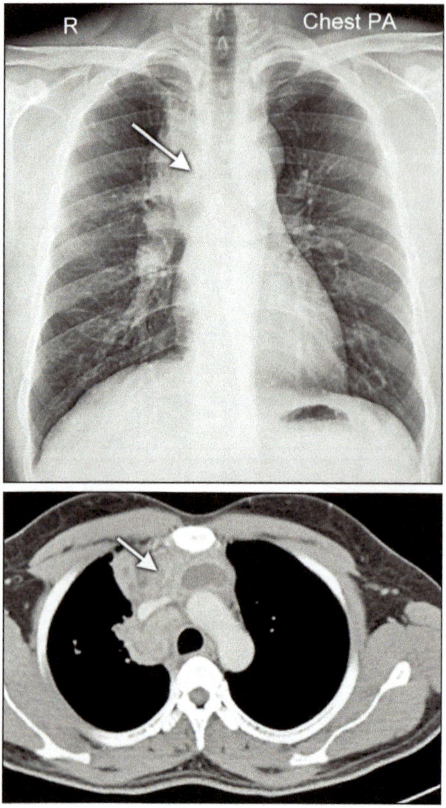

Fig. 5.17: Case 17.

CASE 18

Diagnosis: Bronchiolitis

Chest X-ray shows bilateral ill-defined nodular opacities. HRCT coronal reformats show the nature and distribution of bronchiolar opacities **(Fig. 5.18)**.

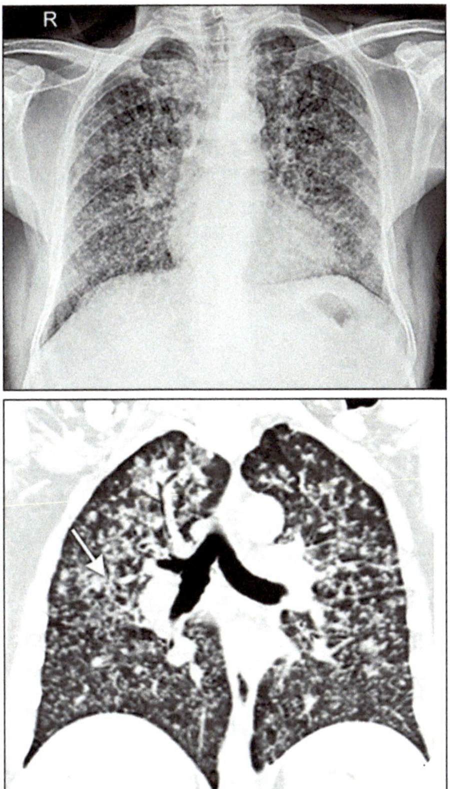

Fig. 5.18: Case 18.

CASE 19

Diagnosis: Infective bronchiolitis—probably Koch's.

Chest X-ray shows right mid-zone nodular opacities. HRCT section shows right upper lobe posterior segment bronchiolar tree in bud appearance **(Fig. 5.19)**.

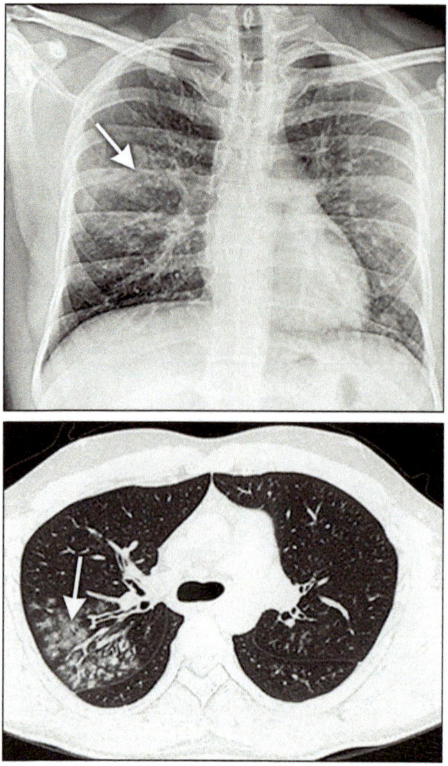

Fig. 5.19: Case 19.

CASE 20

Diagnosis: Healed Koch's lesions.

Chest X-ray shows multiple bilateral high-density opacities with fibrotic changes, CT section shows calcific densities reflecting healed Koch's lesions with sequelae **(Fig. 5.20)**.

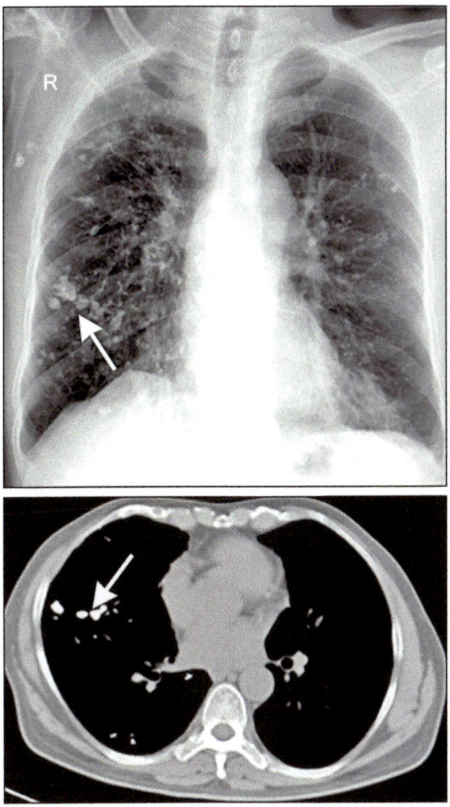

Fig. 5.20: Case 20.

CASE 21

Diagnosis: Retrocardiac bronchiectasis.

Chest X-ray shows left lower zone retrocardiac lucencies, HRCT section shows bronchiectatic changes. CT helps in delineating the correct segmental anatomy and associated complications to help plan treatment **(Fig. 5.21)**.

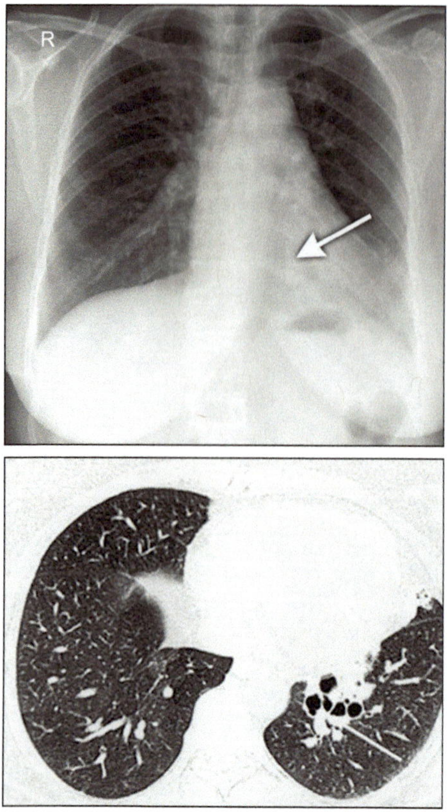

Fig. 5.21: Case 21.

CASE 22

Diagnosis: Right lower zone and middle lobe medial subsegmental atelectasis.

Chest X-ray shows a linear right lower zone and middle lobe opacity, CT sections show the peripheral plate atelectasis with right middle lobe medial segment subsegmental atelectasis **(Fig. 5.22)**.

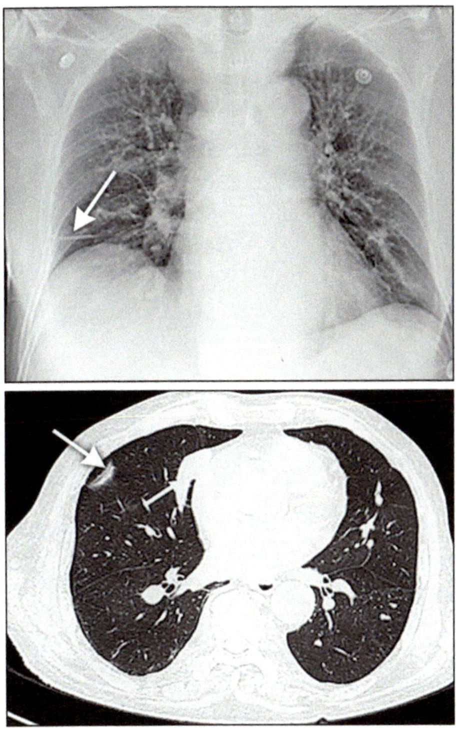

Fig. 5.22: Case 22.

CASE 23

Diagnosis: Cryptogenic organizing pneumonia.

Chest X-ray shows multiple peripheral opacities, HRCT section shows peripheral subpleural consolidation, some of the nodules showed reverse halo sign (arrow) suggesting the diagnosis of COP **(FIG. 5.23)**.

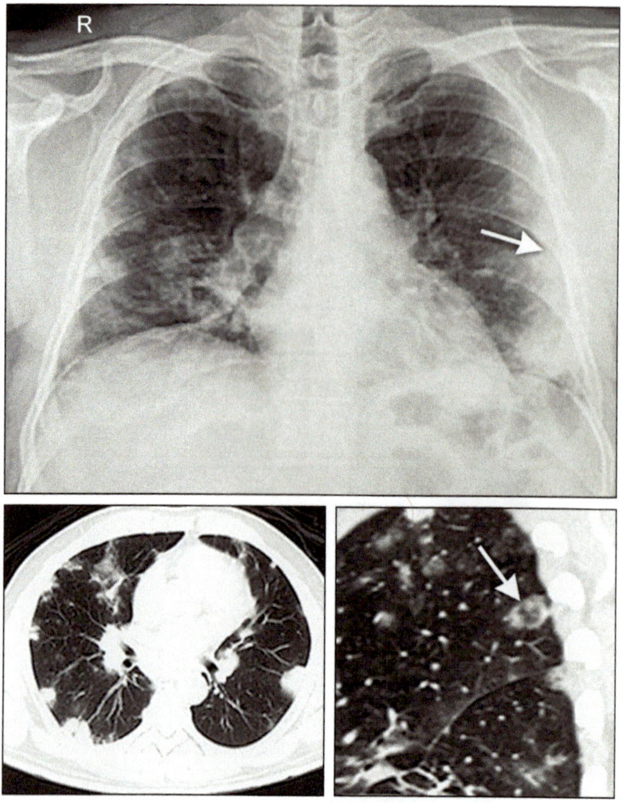

Fig. 5.23: Case 23.

CASE 24

Diagnosis: Metastatic osseous mediastinal node from right humeral osteosarcoma.

Chest X-ray shows right mediastinal calcified node. Right humeral prosthesis is seen (postoperative status osteosarcoma). CT section shows the osseous matrix of the right mediastinal node **(Fig. 5.24)**.

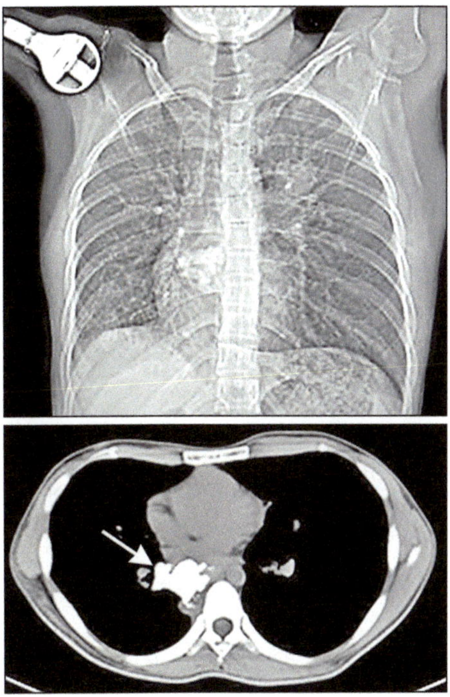

Fig. 5.24: Case 24.

CASE 25

Diagnosis: Massive left pleural effusion.

Chest X-ray shows opaque left hemithorax. CT section shows massive left pleural effusion with underlying passive atelectasis of left lung. CT often helps in diagnosing the cause of opaque hemithorax helping to guide treatment **(Fig. 5.25)**.

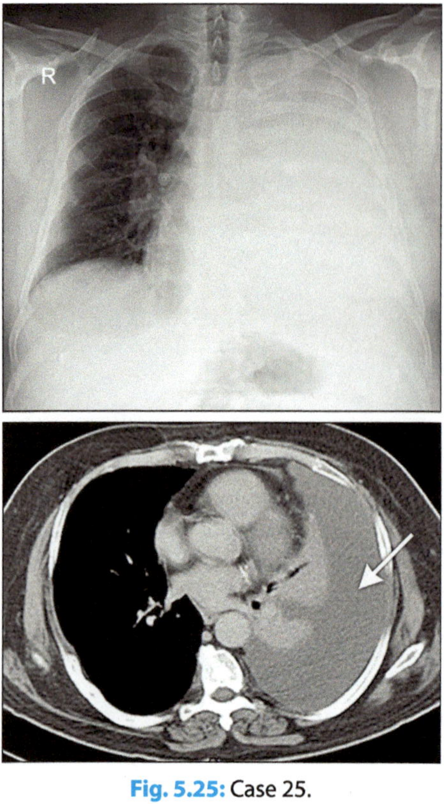

Fig. 5.25: Case 25.

CASE 26

Diagnosis: End-stage left lung.

Chest X-ray shows volume loss of left hemithorax with secondary changes of tracheal and mediastinal shift. Coronal CT sections show the cystic end stage changes of left lung parenchyma with compensatory changes of the right lung. CT helps in surgical planning **(Fig. 5.26)**.

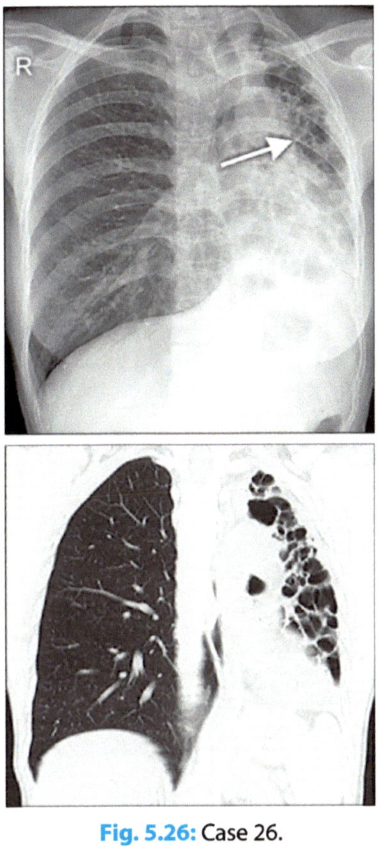

Fig. 5.26: Case 26.

CASE 27

Diagnosis: Right pneumothorax with ICD tube. Right upper lung contusion with laceration and rib fractures.

Chest X-ray shows right pneumothorax with subcutaneous emphysema and ICD, right upper lobe opacity with central lucency and rib fractures. Coronal CT image shows the parenchymal contusion with central lucencies suggesting a diagnosis of associated pulmonary laceration. CT is an extremely useful tool in trauma assessment as it characterizes injuries involving all compartments **(Fig. 5.27)**.

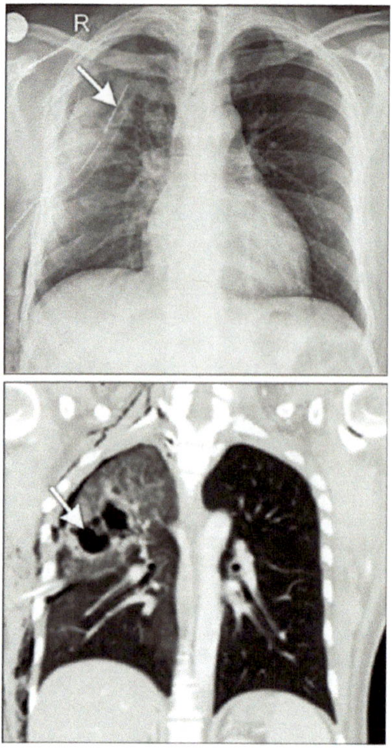

Fig. 5.27: Case 27.

CASE 28

Diagnosis: Left prominent costophrenic fat pad.

Chest X-ray shows a left CP angle opacity obscuring the margins in a febrile patient thought to be pleural effusion, CT section helps in correct diagnosis of fat **(Fig. 5.28)**.

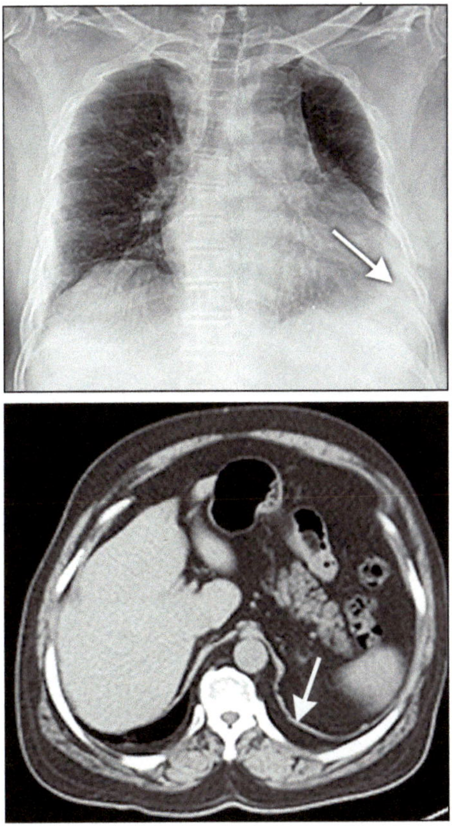

Fig. 5.28: Case 28.

CASE 29

Diagnosis: Lymphangioleiomyomatosis (LAM)

Chest X-ray shows right pneumothorax with bilateral thin-walled lucent opacities. HRCT section shows lung to be replaced by numerous thin-walled cysts with some intervening parenchyma. Right pneumothorax also noted. CT helps in correct diagnosis of LAM **(Fig. 5.29)**.

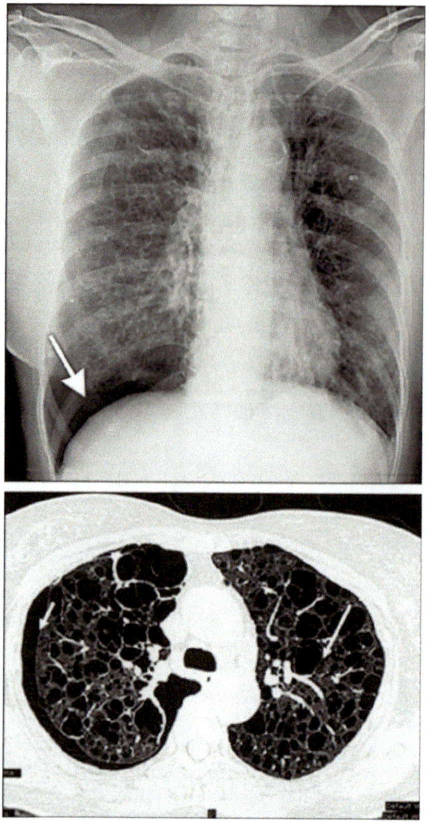

Fig. 5.29: Case 29.

CASE 30

Diagnosis: Left bronchial web with left obstructive emphysema.

Chest X-ray shows lucent left hemithorax. Axial CT helps in the correct diagnosis of left bronchial web. Volume rendered CT image shows hyperinflation of left hemithorax and the left bronchial stenosis **(Fig. 5.30)**.

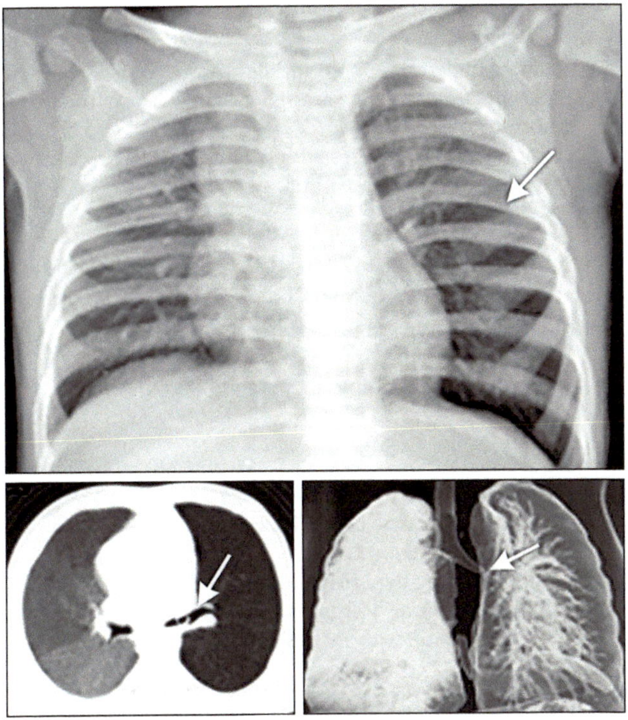

Fig. 5.30: Case 30.

MULTIPLE CHOICE QUESTIONS

1. **A patient's chest X-ray shows multiple peripheral opacities, HRCT section shows peripheral subpleural consolidation, some of the nodules showed reverse halo sign. What is the most probable diagnosis?**
   a. Asbestosis
   b. Lung cancer
   c. Cryptogenic organizing pneumonia (COP)
   d. Pulmonary embolism

2. **What is the characteristic finding on HRCT Thorax in patients with LAM?**
   a. Diffuse bilateral reticulonodular opacities
   b. Multiple thin-walled rounded cysts with or without pneumothorax
   c. Ground-glass opacities with bronchial wall thickening
   d. Mediastinal lymphadenopathy

3. **A patient's chest X-ray shows central bronchiectasis with proximal tubular opacities. HRCT sections at the exact anatomical location shows bronchiectasis with mucoid impaction. What is the probable diagnosis?**
   a. Pneumocystis pneumonia
   b. Allergic bronchopulmonary aspergillosis (ABPA)
   c. Tuberculosis
   d. Histoplasma capsulatum

4. **Which of the following findings is characteristic of Kartagener syndrome on CT imaging?**
   a. Bilateral lower lobe fibrosis
   b. Unilateral lung hyperinflation
   c. Bronchiectasis and situs inversus
   d. Pleural effusion without atelectasis

5. **What pattern of opacities is commonly seen on HRCT in acute extrinsic allergic alveolitis [EAA]?**
   a. Reticular opacities with ground-glass attenuation
   b. Consolidation with air bronchograms

c. Centrilobular nodular opacities
d. Mosaic perfusion pattern

6. Which of the following is a classic finding on chest X-ray in pulmonary microlithiasis?
a. Honeycombing
b. Ground-glass opacities
c. Diffuse bilateral reticulonodular shadows
d. Mediastinal lymphadenopathy

7. On contrast-enhanced CT (CECT) imaging, lymph nodes in Koch's lymphadenopathy typically demonstrate:
a. Homogeneous enhancement
b. Central hypodense nodes with rim enhancement
c. Calcifications
d. Fat attenuation

ANSWERS

1. c	2. b	3. b	4. c
5. c	6. c	7. b	

CHAPTER 6

Imaging in COVID-19

INTRODUCTION

Coronavirus or novel coronavirus termed as SARS-CoV-2 and named by the World Health Organization (WHO) as COVID-19 emerged from Wuhan city, Hubei Province of China by the end of 2019 and has caused pandemic. SARS-CoV-2 is primarily transmitted between people through respiratory (droplet and aerosol) and contact routes. Risk of transmission is highest where people are in close proximity (within 2 meters). In healthcare settings where procedures or support treatments that generate aerosols are performed, airborne transmission can occur. Poorly ventilated indoor spaces increase the chances of transmission by air, particularly if individuals are in the same room together for an extended period.

Clinical Features

COVID-19 presents with a range of symptoms of varying severity. Asymptomatic infection also occurs often although frequency is not defined.

More common symptoms are: Fever, new and continuous cough, shortness of breath, fatigue, loss of appetite, anosmia (loss of smell), ageusia (loss of taste).

Non-specific symptoms include: Shortness of breath, fatigue, loss of appetite, myalgia, sore throat, headache, nasal congestion, diarrhea, nausea, vomiting.

Atypical symptoms, such as delirium and reduced mobility, can present in older and immunocompromised people, often in the absence of a fever.

Assessment and Diagnosis (Table 6.1)

Reverse transcription polymerase chain reaction-based SARS-CoV-2 RNA detection from respiratory samples (e.g. nasopharynx) is the standard for diagnosis.

HRCT thorax is highly sensitive but has low specificity.

TABLE 6.1: CO-RADS: Level of suspicion of COVID-19 infection.

	Suspicion	*CT findings*
CO-RADS 1	No	Normal or noninfectious abnormalities
CO-RADS 2	Low	Abnormalities consistent with infections other than COVID-19
CO-RADS 3	Indeterminate	Unclear whether COVID-19 is present
CO-RADS 4	High	Abnormalities suspicious for COVID-19
CO-RADS 5	Very high	Typical COVID-19
CO-RADS 6	PCR+	

Approaches to Imaging

A dedicated route for radiological investigations is established. If imaging is to be done with portable equipment (chest or abdominal radiography), the technologist dons PPE and performs portable radiography in the isolation room. PPE consists of a gown, gloves, eye protection, and a mask. Once radiographic scan is complete, the technologist doffs PPE gear, preferably with a trained observer monitoring removal, ensures that the patient continues to wear a mask and will direct the patient out of the department. Air disinfection is done before starting the scan and after its completion.

Imaging (Figs. 6.1 to 6.3)

Typical chest X-ray findings of COVID-19 are multifocal, bilateral (>unilateral) radiopacities with lower lung and peripheral predominance.

Atypical chest X-ray findings of COVID-19 are pleural effusion, pneumothorax, cavitation, solitary/diffuse lung nodule.

Chest computed tomographic imaging abnormalities for COVID-19 are multifocal, bilateral (>unilateral), basal and peripheral distribution of ground-glass opacities with or without consolidation. Ground-glass opacities may have

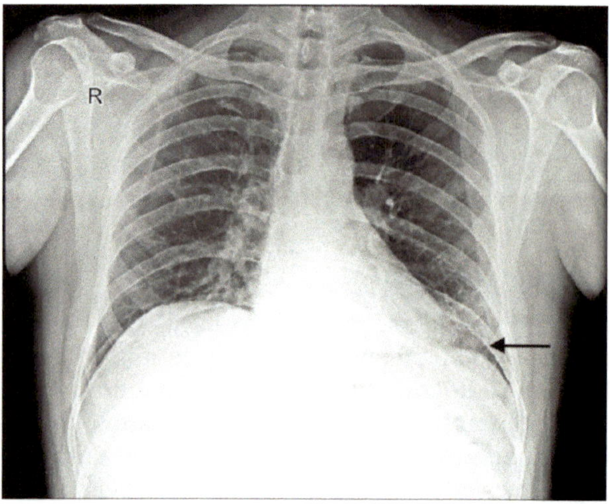

Fig. 6.1: CXR AP view shows subtle haze (arrow) in left lower lung field. Findings are likely suggestive of mild pulmonary involvement.

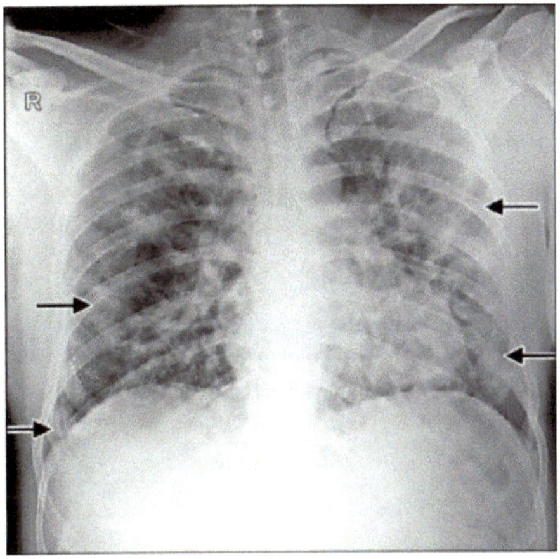

Fig. 6.2: CXR AP view shows multiple ground glass opacities (arrows) noted in bilateral lung fields with peripheral predominance. Findings are likely suggestive of moderate to severe pulmonary involvement.

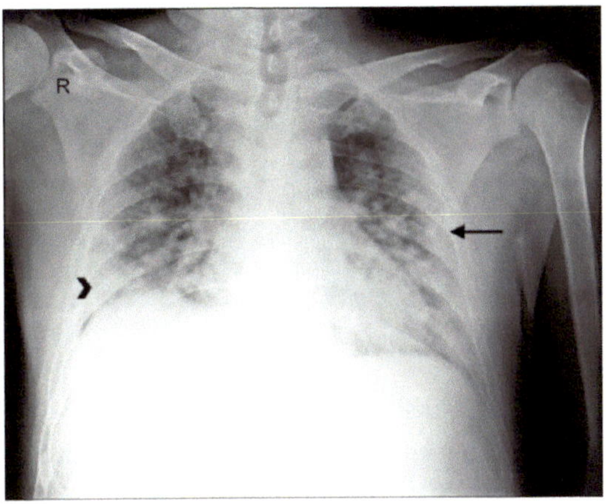

Fig. 6.3: CXR AP view shows multiple ground glass opacities (arrow) in bilateral lung fields with area of consolidation in right lower lung field (arrowhead). Findings are likely suggestive of severe pulmonary involvement.

ill-defined margins, air bronchograms, smooth or irregular interlobular thickening or intralobular lines giving crazy paving pattern, traction bronchiectasis, vascular dilatation, subpleural bands and architectural distortion.

CT involvement score is given by scoring the percentage of involvement of each of five (maximum score 25) lobes as follows **(Tables 6.2 and 6.3)**:

TABLE 6.2: Score with respect to lung involvement.

Score	*Lung involvement*
0	Absent
1	<5%
2	5–25%
3	25–50%
4	50–75%
5	>75%

TABLE 6.3: Interpretation of the pulmonary involvement.

Score	*Pulmonary involvement*
<8	Mild
9–15	Moderate
>15	Severe

POST-COVID-19 SEQUELAE

1. Fibrosis
2. Mucormycosis

CASE: Characteristic chest radiograph finding in a 44-year-old male presenting with cough, fever and breathlessness for 4 days **(Fig. 6.4)**.

Chest radiographic finding includes bilateral patchy and confluent, band-like ground-glass and consolidative opacities showing peripheral distribution involving middle to lower lung zones.

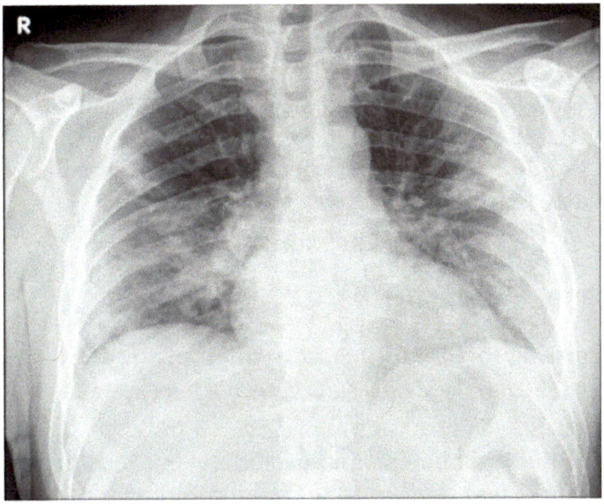

Fig. 6.4: Chest X-ray PA view in a COVID-19 patient.

MULTIPLE CHOICE QUESTIONS

1. **What is the severity score of a mild case of COVID-19 infection on HRCT thorax?**
   a. 0 b. 1–8
   c. 9–15 d. 16–25

2. **What is the severity score of a moderate case of COVID-19 infection on HRCT thorax?**
   a. 0 b. 1–8
   c. 9–15 d. 16–25

3. **What is the severity score of a severe case of COVID-19 infection on HRCT thorax?**
   a. >25 b. 1–8
   c. 9–15 d. 16–25

4. **What is the typical pattern on chest X-ray of a COVID-19 pneumonia patient?**
   a. Bilateral and peripheral
   b. Unilateral

c. Bilateral and asymmetrical
d. Any of the above

5. **Which of the following CT features is frequently observed in COVID-19 pneumonia?**
   a. Multifocal ground glass opacities (GGO) with peripheral distribution
   b. Consolidations
   c. Pericardial effusion
   d. Pleural effusions

6. **According to US Multicenter which of the following is not a typical pattern on chest X-ray of a COVID-19 infected patient?**
   a. Multifocal bilateral and peripheral predominance
   b. Bilateral and lower zones predominant
   c. Bilateral and upper zones predominant
   d. None

7. **Which of the following is a post-COVID-19 sequelae?**
   a. Fibrotic changes in lungs
   b. Mucormycosis
   c. Traction bronchiectasis changes in lung
   d. All of the above

8. **Who are at risk for death with COVID-19 pneumonia?**
   a. Cardiac diseases
   b. Age >60 years
   c. Diabetes, TB, HIV and chronic diseases
   d. All of the above

9. **What precautions will you take while managing a confirmed COVID-19 case?**
   a. Use PPE (medical mask, eye protection, gloves and gown) when entering room and remove PPE when leaving
   b. Avoid contaminating environmental surfaces (e.g., door handles and light switches)
   c. Ensure adequate room ventilation
   d. All of the above

10. What are the elements of standard precautions while handling COVID-19 case?
   a. Hand hygiene and respiratory hygiene
   b. PPE (personal protective equipment) according to the risk
   c. Safe injection practices, sharps management and injury prevention, safe handling, cleaning and disinfection of patient care equipment
   d. All of the above

ANSWERS

1. b	2. c	3. d	4. a
5. a	6. d	7. d	8. d
9. d.	10. d		

Appendices

APPENDIX 1: CHEST X-RAY—BASICS

REVIEW OF NORMAL CHEST

In many ways the skills needed to look at diagnostic radiographs are the same ones used for performing physical examinations on patients. For example, careful observation of findings coupled with a systematic review of systems are the same in both.

Get in the habit of always checking the following items before anything else. It takes a few seconds and is an important legal safeguard as well.

- Patient's name.
- Date examination done (very important if comparing prior exams)
- Check for position markers—right vs. left, upright. Other items to check before commencing with clinical review of the film include:
- Patient's position—supine, upright, lateral, decubitus
- Technical quality of examination—learn what are the acceptable limits for the examination. You cannot find a subtle pneumothorax if there is patient motion or the film is overexposed.

INITIAL SURVEY

- General body size, shape, and symmetry
- Male vs. female
- Is this an infant, child, young adult, elderly person?
- Survey for foreign objects—tubes, IV lines, electrocardiography (ECG) leads, surgical drains, prosthesis, etc., as well as nonmedical objects, bullets, shrapnel, glass, etc.

SOFT TISSUES AND SKELETAL STRUCTURE (FIG. A.1)

Soft tissues—look again at overall amount, then check for the following: calcifications, obvious mass effect, abnormal air collections (called subcutaneous emphysema), and soft tissue companion shadow for the clavicle (this is a normal but variable finding).

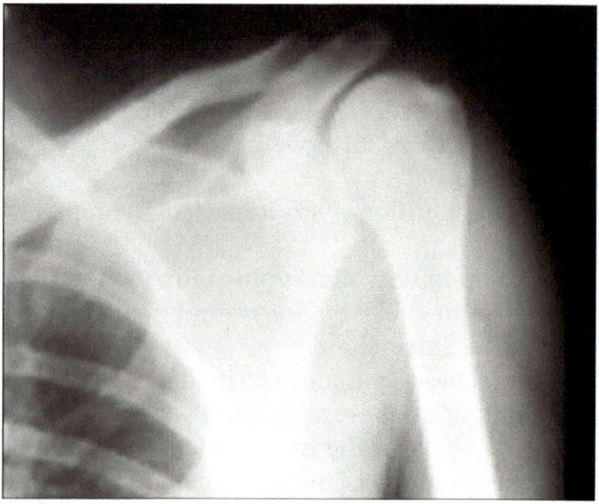

Fig. A.1: X-ray of shoulder girdle - bones and soft tissues.

Bones—look at each bone for the following items (notice again the progression from general to increasingly specific detail throughout the review).

- Overall size, shape, and contour of each bone
- The density or mineralization
- Compare cortical thickness to medullary cavity, trabecular pattern, look for erosions, fractures, any lytic or blastic regions
- At joints, are articular relationships normal, joint spaces narrowed, widened, any calcification in the cartilages, air in the joint space, abnormal fat pads, etc.

CHEST WALL (FIG. A.2)

Look for overall thickness, subcutaneous emphysema, calcification. Look for sharp, distinct borders.

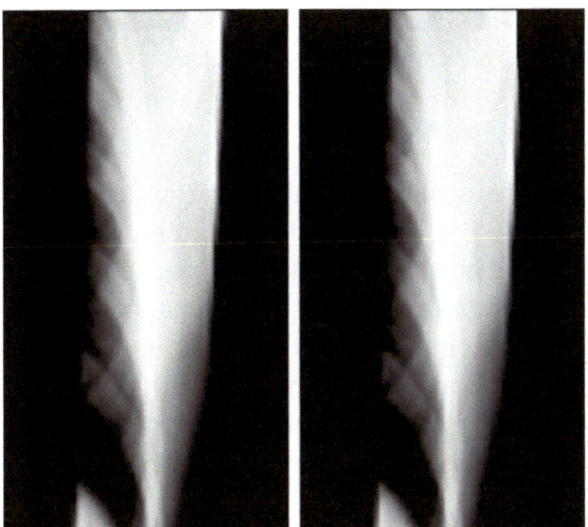

Fig. A.2: Chest wall with ribs.

BREAST TISSUE (FIG. A.3)

In males and females, some asymmetry can occur from standing with unequal pressure against the film holder. Notice how the apparent lung density changes from the lung area covered by the soft tissue of the breast to the lung area inferior to the breast.

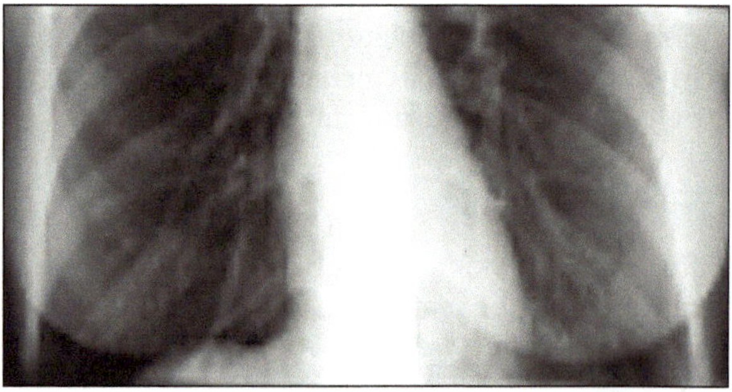

Fig. A.3: Breast shadow.

ABDOMEN (FIG. A.4)

The visibility of structures is highly variable but look for the following even if you see very few on any one exam.

- Gastric and bowel gas—is amount and location normal?
- Check for organ size of liver, spleen, and kidneys if visible.
- Check for free peritoneal air—remember position of patient will change location of free air.
- Look for calcifications and masses—can they be localized to a specific structure.

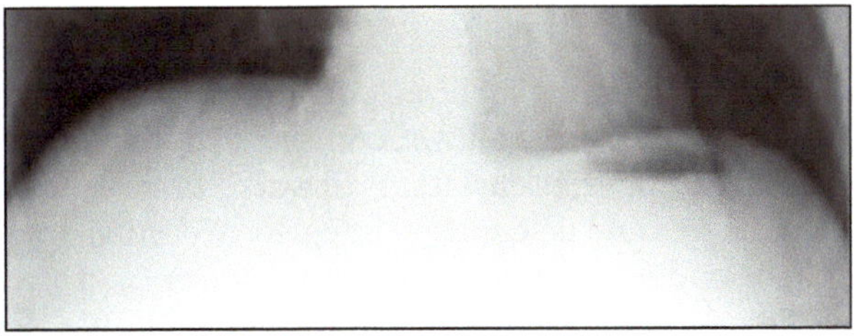

Fig. A.4: Diaphragm and gastric air bubble.

NECK SOFT TISSUES AND SPINE (FIG. A.5)

Check overall amounts of soft tissue, presence of calcifications, subcutaneous emphysema, position and size of trachea. For the cervical spine, check alignment and note any major congenital abnormalities. Then look at specific parts of the vertebra and disc spaces, checking for erosions, lytic or blastic lesions, disc and synovial joint narrowing or other abnormalities.

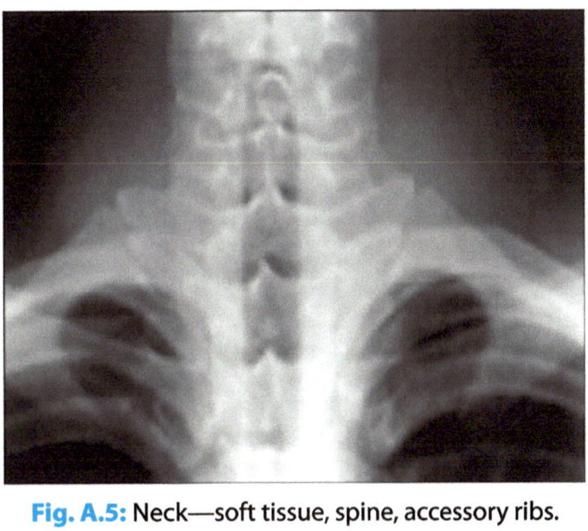

Fig. A.5: Neck—soft tissue, spine, accessory ribs.

THORACIC SPINE (FIG. A.6)

Look at specific parts of each vertebra and the disc spaces as far caudally as the image allows, compare frontal and lateral projections. Some check list items to watch for are: height of vertebral bodies and disc spaces, integrity of cortical margins around the bodies, pedicles, and lamina, presence of any lytic or sclerotic areas, normal spacing of synovial joints, versus narrowing or sclerosis.

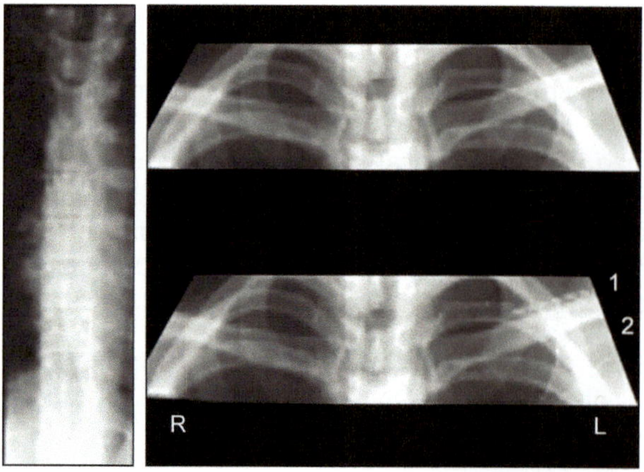

Fig. A.6: Thoracic spine, paravertebral stripes.

RIBS

Compare individual ribs side to side, check specific parts, cortical margins, trabecular patterns. Make a note if the anterior cartilages are calcified, frequently the first one does so irregularly and may obscure or mimic underlying lung lesions.

- Posterior rib
- Anterior rib

SUPERIOR MEDIASTINUM—POSTEROANTERIOR (FIG. A.7)

First, check the overall width for normal size, again look for masses, calcifications, and free air. The rest of the superior mediastinum review is a detailed search for subtle distortion of several major pleural mediastinal interfaces.

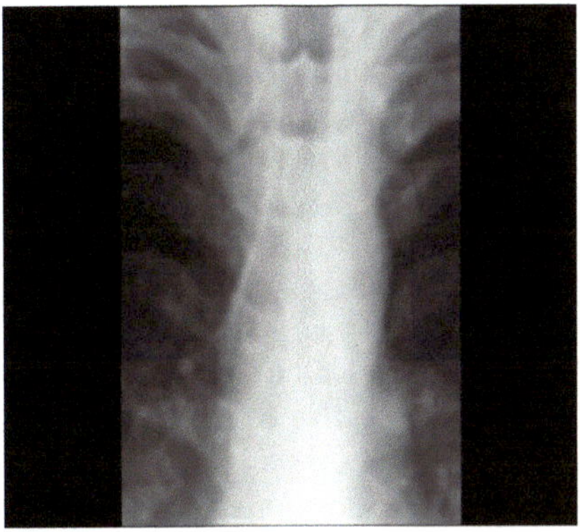

Fig. A.7: Superior mediastinal planes.

MARGIN OF SUPERIOR VENA CAVA

The superior vena cava (SVC) is seen on the frontal view only, and depending how laterally it projects, its right edge may cast a subtle line on the film. Sometimes the entire edge is seen, often only a portion, but it should not bulge into the lung with a convex border.

RIGHT PARATRACHEAL STRIPE

The normal width is less than 5 mm, usually it is only 2–3 mm. This is an important marker for otherwise subtle adenopathy. The distal end of the stripe is formed by the azygos vein, and if the vein is distended, that portion of the stripe may normally be up to 1 cm wide. The medial margin of the stripe is the air-soft tissue interface along the right mucosal surface of the trachea. The outer margin of the stripe begins around the level of the medial end of the clavicle and is formed by the pleural surface of the right upper lobe (RUL) against the mediastinum. The only structures normally at that level to give soft tissue density between the air filled trachea and the RUL are the right wall of the trachea, nerves, some fat, lymph nodes, and pleura of the RUL. The stripe ends where the RUL bronchus sweeps under the azygos vein as the latter arches anteriorly to empty into the posterior surface of the SVC.

LEFT SUBCLAVIAN STRIPE

The normal width is 1.0–1.5 cm. Its inner margin is the air mucosal interface along the left mucosal surface of the trachea, and its outer margin is the interface of the medial aspect of the left upper lobe against the lateral margin of the left subclavian artery. You usually will pick up the outer edge of the stripe at the level of the clavicle and will be able to follow it down to the bulge of the aortic arch.

Anterior Middle and Posterior Mediastinum

Review the heart for overall size and shape. A rough yardstick for size on the frontal film is the ratio of the widest diameter of the heart to the widest width of the thoracic cage as measured from inner aspect of rib to rib. This cardiac-thoracic ratio should be less than 50% (see inset for a graphic illustration of ratio measurements). Look carefully for calcifications, pneumopericardium, pneumomediastinum, sutures, prosthetic valves, etc. that you may have overlooked on the general survey of the entire mediastinum.

AORTA

Try tracking it from the root to distal descending aorta. In the young adult the ascending aorta usually is hidden in the mediastinum, in older people it may swing to the right enough to cast a soft tissue bulge. The arch should always be seen, make sure it is to the left of the distal trachea and actually pushes the distal trachea slightly to the right. Check for aortic calcifications and size. The left lateral border of the descending aorta abuts the left lung.

PULMONARY ARTERY

On the frontal view, the only part of the main pulmonary artery seen is the left lateral border where it meets the left lung. It can be relatively straight or convex (most commonly in young females). When convex, it forms a "middle mogul" just above the heart. The upper "mogul" is the aortic knob, the lower mogul is the left ventricle. The left pulmonary artery is directly behind the main pulmonary artery, and is visible on frontal films as a branching structure.

AZYGOESOPHAGEAL LINE OR PARAESOPHAGEAL LINE

This is seen on the frontal view only and is formed by the right lower lobe where it meets the portion of the mediastinum containing the esophagus and the azygos vein. It usually overlies the thoracic spine, at or near the midline, and is usually fairly straight, vertically. If it bulges convex toward the lung, be suspicious of a mediastinal mass, usually subcarinal lymph nodes or an enlarged left atrium.

RIGHT AND LEFT PULMONARY ARTERIES

On the frontal view, the left pulmonary artery is the soft tissue density behind the main pulmonary artery, branching into the lung. The proximal right pulmonary artery is buried in the mediastinum, and is not seen on the frontal view until it branches as the right hilum.

PULMONARY ARTERIES, LATERAL VIEW

The right pulmonary artery is seen on the lateral view as an ovoid branching structure, just anterior to the air column of the trachea and main bronchi. The left pulmonary artery is never seen as clearly as the right, unless it is markedly enlarged. It is a curved shadow, similar in shape to the aorta, just behind the air column.

AORTICOPULMONARY WINDOW (AP WINDOW)

This is another area radiologists double check for subtle mediastinal masses. It is seen on the frontal view (line of white dots) and is formed by a portion of the upper lobe sitting in the space immediately lateral to the area between the aortic arch and left pulmonary artery (remember ligamentum arteriosum and left recurrent laryngeal nerve?). The AP window should have a concave or straight border. If there is a mediastinal mass in the AP window region, the lung will be pushed laterally and the border becomes convex.

PARASPINAL EDGES (STRIPES)

Sometimes on the frontal view, the pleural edge is seen as a vertical density running parallel to the lateral margins of the vertebral bodies. If visible, this edge should be only a few millimeters beyond the vertebral bodies, and should not be lumpy or bulging (The paraspinal edges are not visible on this image).

APPENDIX 2: HILA

FRONTAL VIEW OF THE HILA

As visible on the frontal view, most of the hilar shadows are the left and right pulmonary arteries. The bronchi run with the arteries, but are, of course, lucent. The pulmonary veins are not clearly seen because they are behind the widest parts of the heart, inferior to the hila, where they converge into the left atrium. The left pulmonary artery is always more superior than the right, thus making the left hilum appear higher. Calcified lymph nodes may be visible within the hilar shadows.

PARENCHYMA

Large abnormalities will have already been seen, but now is the time to search carefully for small masses, infiltrates, calcifications, etc. Compare small sections of lung side to side at a time. Use the same techniques as you used for comparing ribs but now ignore the bone and look at the lung. There are three areas in which small lung lesions are easily overlooked: behind the calcified anterior first rib cartilage, behind the heart, and behind the diaphragm.

LATERAL VIEW OF THE LUNG (FIG. A.8)

The lateral view is your great chance to look at the lung in the posterior costophrenic recess and anterior mediastinum.

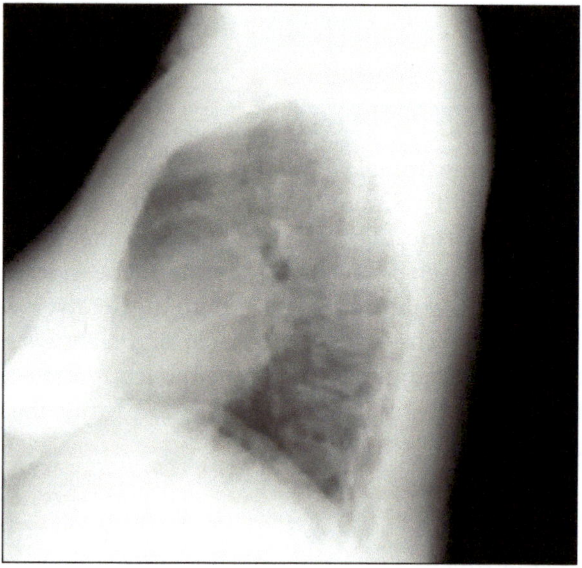

Fig. A.8: Chest X-ray lateral view.

PLEURA

Check the frontal view for minor fissure thickness and location, and on the lateral view, look for minor and major fissures even if you do not see them in their entirety which you rarely will. These are normally fine delicate structures that do not show up on the digitized images.

Checklist

- Check patient name, position, technical quality.
- Soft tissue including breast, chest wall, companion shadow.
- Review soft tissues and skeletal structures of shoulder girdles and chest wall.

- Review abdomen for bowel gas, organ size, abnormal calcifications, free air, etc.
- Review soft tissues and spine of neck.
- Review spine and rib cage—check alignment, disk space narrowing, lytic or blastic regions, etc.
- Review mediastinum:
  - Overall size and shape
  - Trachea—position
  - Margins—SVC, ascending aorta, right atrium, left subclavian artery, aortic arch, main pulmonary artery, left ventricle
  - Lines and stripes—paratracheal, paraspinal, para-esophageal (azygoesophageal), para-aortic
  - Retrosternal clear space.
- Review hila:
  - Normal relationships
  - Size.
- Review lungs and pleura:
  - Compare lung sizes
  - Evaluate pulmonary vascular pattern—compare upper to lower lobe, right to left, normal tapering to periphery
  - Pulmonary parenchyma
  - Pleural surfaces
    - Fissures—major and minor, if seen
    - Compare hemidiaphragms
    - Follow pleura around rib cage.

Index

Page numbers followed by *f* refer to figure and *t* refer to table

D

I

K

L

S

T

U

V

W

X